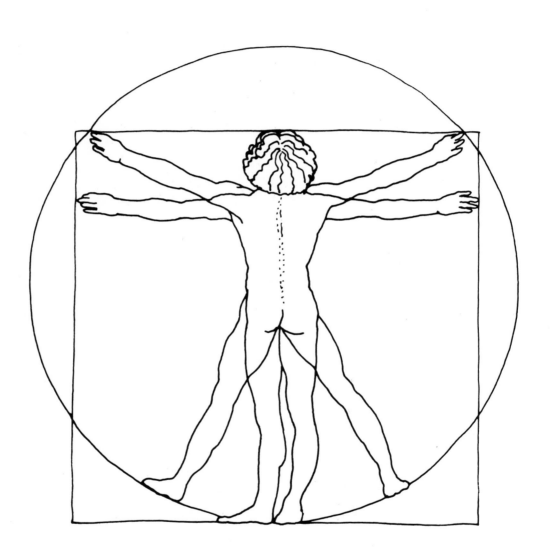

# THE
# BASIC
# BACK BOOK

**Anne Kent Rush**

MOON BOOKS/SUMMIT BOOKS

Cover design: Freude
Cover concept & illustration: Anne Kent Rush
Book design & illustrations: Anne Kent Rush
First printing: August, 1979
Typeset at Ann Flanagan Typography, Berkeley
Production: Margit Stange
Text type: Century Old Style
Co-published by: Moon Books and Summit Books (A Simon & Schuster Division of Gulf & Western Corporation)
Moon Books, Box 9223, Berkeley, California 94709
Summit Books, Simon & Schuster, 1230 Avenue of the Americas, New York, N.Y. 10020
Distributed by Simon & Schuster, Inc.

Other Moon Books titles: THE KIN OF ATA, Dorothy Bryant: MOON, MOON, Anne Kent Rush; FROM A SPANISH PRISON, Eva Forest; THE GREAT SIOUX NATION, Roxanne Dunbar Oritz; BLOOD TIES, Anica Vesel Mander; THE NEW LESBIANS, Covina & Galana; TOWARD A NEW EXPRESSION, S. Santoro; LOST GODDESSES OF EARLY GREECE, Charlene Spretnak; INTERVIEW WITH THE MUSE, Nina Winter. All Moon Books can be single copy ordered from WIND, Box 8858, Washington D.C. 20003

Library of Congress Cataloging in Publication Data

Rush, Anne Kent, date.
  The basic back book.

  "A Moon book."
  1. Backache. I. Title.
RD768.R87        617'.5        79-15651
ISBN 0-671-40055-X
ISBN 0-671-40086-X pbk.
Manufactured in the U.S.A.

*Publisher's Note*

This book contains certain exercises and suggested procedures to aid in preventing back problems. It does not make any specific medical recommendations. Any person experiencing a back problem should consult with a physician prior to engaging in any of the exercises or procedures.

# Acknowledgments

I would like to thank especially my editor, Stephanie Mills, my researcher, Jan Navsky, and my typist, Barbara Corso, without whose fine work this book would not have been done in any reasonable time or condition. Andy Gillin also deserves thanks for asking me to produce the original pamphlet out of which the idea for this book came. Freude contributed her graphic and editorial skills in invaluable ways. Christine Steinmetz and Jim Silberman of Summit continued their encouragement of my work. My uncle Norton and my parents in Alabama urged me on in the ways only a family can. Moussla took my burdens on her back when I needed to forsake typewriters for grassy fields. The support of many other friends and of the contributors also helped make putting together this book a rich process. And Tahiti provided perspective on beauty and pleasure, to reaffirm my knowledge that happiness is the best back doctor.

# Contents

# Note

Throughout the text I have sprinkled the words "they" or "their" where strict grammar would demand the singular pronoun. I chose to sacrifice grammar in my attempt to avoid using the words "he" or "his" when referring to the individual in a world composed of at least equal numbers of "shes" and "hers." Because I hope this book will be useful to both women and men this priority seems reasonable, although it may cause a few readers some confusion. Well, we are all in the soup together and are still seeking a practical solution, along with A.A. Milne, who, in POOH'S BIRTHDAY BOOK, said "If the English language had been properly organized . . . then there would be a word which meant both "he" and "she," and I could write, 'If John or Mary comes, heesh will want to play tennis,' which would save a lot of trouble."[1]

# I
# Beginning

# Why A Back Book?

Everybody has a back, and nearly everybody has back troubles. According to a recent United States Public Health Service report, more people contract back problems at some time during their lives than any other medical ailment.

A common explanation of this fact is "Human beings were never meant to walk on two legs." No doubt if we walked on all fours we could release the downward pressure that is the blight of many spines. However, we humans seem determined to walk upright and to do all kinds of things that our backs were probably never "meant to do."

We need to learn to integrate activities into our daily lives which counteract the strains of modern living and keep us from suffering chronic aches, or from resorting to debilitating and painful solutions like drugs and surgery. Except in rare and urgent cases, I am against surgery for back and neck injuries. Most doctors will tell you that the success rate of operations for common back problems is usually the same as the success rate of rest and exercise treatments. When there is a choice, surgery should be the last resort, because such treatments often compound the trauma to our bodies rather than heal them.

Over my years of experience studying and working in various forms of body therapies, I have arrived at an alternative approach to healing our backs. The exercises in this book are based on the idea that healing takes place most effectively through pleasure and relaxation. My studies in physical therapies included work in Reichian, Proskauer, Breyer, Feldenkrais, Alexander, massage, and Polarity techniques; and I spent three years on the Esalen Institute staff conducting training programs in Polarity Therapy for health professionals. During my years in private practice as a body therapist I worked with clients who had many types of back and neck disorders. Except for those resulting from accidents, the problems were almost entirely caused by a simple combination of physical and psychological tension: bad posture and emotional stress. These are causes which we can treat ourselves by changing our habits and by becoming more sensitive to our responses to our environment.

The back experts interviewed in this book define many causes and treatments of back problems. No matter how diverse their approaches to treatment, they all agree that the three critical origins of back problems are: stress, inappropriate diet, and lack of proper exercise. Stress, emotional or physical, is the single most critical factor to consider because even with good diet and proper exercise our health can be undermined by stress. We must take care to alternate work or pressured periods with relaxation. Diet is also critical because what we eat is what our bodies become made of. If we do not eat well, after years of straining to transform chemicals into the proper substances, our systems will give out. On the other hand if we eat well consistently our bodies will have the fuel to maintain optimum tone and chemical balance at any age. Proper and regular exercise is the third ingredient of good back care. Too rough or too much exercise can produce as many problems as too little. Learning to move well throughout a normal day's activities can reduce your need for separate exercise periods. Teaching you to move well is the aim of the exercises in this book.

THE BASIC BACK BOOK can be used by anyone of any age who wants to learn preventive measures to ward off back problems, or to relieve back pain caused by accident, illness, or bad habits. There are sections on preventive exercises, exercises for conditions after injury, and treatments for emergency injuries. THE BASIC BACK BOOK covers neck as well as back stress, as the neck is the top of the spine and must be attended to in order to treat the rest of the back. Though THE BASIC BACK BOOK includes massage as well as exercises which two or more people can do together, the focus of the book is on self-treatment, which is the most inexpensive and enduring solution to physical imbalance.

Today most people accept the premise that health problems are the result of both physical and psychological causes. And the omniscience of traditional Western medicine is openly questioned. More and more people are turning toward alternative medicines and self-treatment. Holistic medicine is a form developed in response to these changing attitudes toward medical treatment. Doctors at holistic centers believe that a health problem may be caused by a variety of factors in a person's life and so to heal an injury, the whole person must be healed. Clinics where a patient can consult experts from a variety of fields who prescribe several approaches to a problem are opening in many communities. Multiple treatment is an improvement over one track diagnosis which rarely takes the whole human being into account. Long term permanent healing, however, can only be accomplished by positive changes in one's daily life.

Good physical condition is the best preventive medicine. Injuries usually occur at weak points in one's body. Once injured, an area needs special care to bring it up to par with the rest of your body. It's important to maintain a preventive exercise-healing routine even after you are functioning normally. These routines can be very short if necessary. The crucial ingredient is setting aside moments each day to regain your physical/emotional balance. Establishing these habits is often the toughest part of body maintenance. The chapter called "Habit Forming" deals with this dilemma.

The most successful treatments of back and neck injuries are various forms of pleasure-oriented physical therapy and self-healing. These methods focus on relaxing the injured tissue so it settles into its proper place and then on gradually rebuilding its strength and tone through gentle movements. Anxiety and tension are built into our modern lives. Moments of relaxation and sensitivity are the best antidotes. Nothing helps a traumatized nerve or muscle relax into place like pleasure. Medical science has developed theories from neurological research on alternative and stronger sensation dominance over pain which explain aspects of this phenomenon and on the functioning of healing chemicals in our bodies called enkephalins. The back responds to treatments that are really treats. THE BASIC BACK BOOK describes many back revitalizing processes. You can choose the ones which fit your particular condition.

The mental state of healing is the opposite of the states of stress and force. Replacing surgery, medication and manipulation, the long lasting aspects of healing are relaxation, sensitivity, and allowing your body to return to its own balance. These are the new experts. The most effective solutions to our physical aches and limits come when we begin to add preventive habits to our lives outside the doctors' offices, when we think of healing less as a professional mystique, and more as a way of life.

# What Is Health?

You ought not to attempt to cure the eyes without the head, or the head without the body . . . the body without the soul . . . for the part can never be well unless the whole is well.[2]

—Plato; c. 399 B.C.

Health is a state of complete physical, mental and social well-being and not merely the absence of disease or infirmity.[3]

—*Preamble,* Constitution of the World Health Organization, 1946

One thing I always knew how to do: enjoy life. If I have any genius it is a genius for living.[4]

Errol Flynn, MY WICKED, WICKED WAYS

An exciting and new movement is taking place within the medical profession and among lay people: the health movement. The battle, rather than being "against disease," is "for health." This shift in focus changes not only scientific medicine, but also our daily lives. In the fifties few doctors thought of holistic diagnoses or preventive programs, and few joggers were whizzing down the streets.

Western medicine as we know it today, scientific medicine dominated by the search for disease, is a relatively recent phenomenon. Only a century ago, around 1870, Pasteur's discovery that micro-organisms caused critical illness was accepted as a breakthrough in medicine. Thus pathology, which had been a small branch of medical research came to dominate the field and eventually became the definition of medicine itself. Scientists, doctors and lay people were overwhelmed by the immense variety of tiny potential enemies to our health lurking in every breeze and substance of our environment.

Not only did this one branch of medicine predominate, but with it the concept of germs as the single source of health problems. In the past thousands of years lay varied philosophies of health which dealt with the multiplicity of causes of unhealth: climate, individual resistance levels, economic situations, community conditions, personality traits, professional conditions, age, diet, and sex. But enthusiasm for the germ theory led to a monocausal interpretation of health problems and to a denial of the wisdom of other more eclectic healing traditions.

World War II had a side effect in changing this monocausal concept of illness. During the war thousands of Americans and Europeans travelled and lived in climates and situations where their experiences challenged their beliefs about the causes of disease. It became clear that health services and conditions in poor communities and countries were vastly different from those in rich communities. Also prisoners of war, refugees, and diplomats all suffered from health problems which could not simply be diagnosed as having been caused by germs alone. Cultural and political factors became recognized as influences on health which were quite as powerful as bacteria. The ideology of disease and the definition of health were overhauled and broadened, taking wartime experience into account. At this time the World Health Organization drafted its Constitution. The United Nations Technical Preparatory Committee, composed of sixteen M.D.'s from different countries, met in the spring of 1946 in Paris. Its official definition of health was distinguished from the formerly prevailing "absence of disease" philosophy to encompass "a person's complete physical, mental and social well-being."

In the years since this official post war redefinition of health, the practice of medicine has been catching up with an expanded theory. The new medicine emerging today is not a rejection of the valuable advances of scientific medicine, but a re-integration of the social, cultural, and ecological dimensions of health. This more balanced trend of medicine takes the view that there is no health problem with only one cause; every aspect of a person and her or his environment should be taken into account in order to make a responsible diagnosis and prescription.

The category "sick" was also overhauled. Unrealistic and rigid delineations like "handicapped," "sick" and "healthy" were thrown out and a more accurate picture of health as being a continuous scale of strength and weakness in various aspects of being was accepted. No one is one hundred percent functional and healthy; everyone is in some way "handicapped." Health and disease are relative states and for effective use their conceptual frameworks should be dynamic rather than static.

Attributing absolute wisdom to physicians, nurses, and other official health workers has also given way to a more eclectic attitude on the part of most doctors and lay people. Not only are treatments of other professionals such as psychologists, nutritionists and vocational therapists granted to be of potential healing value to an individual with a health problem, but individuals themselves are seen as crucially responsible for their own cures. Many of these "advances" in medical thinking are actually revivals of ancient systems of health and philosophy. We are being encouraged once again to see our health in terms of our entire being, our total development and our place in the cultural environment.

\*   \*   \*

**You have heard of the Four Medicine Arrows that were brought to us by Sweet Medicine? . . . Every story is meant to be unfolded from each of the Four Great Ways. From the directions of Wisdom, Innocence, Sees Far, and Look-Within . . . The Medicine points the Way for man to learn about himself, his brother, the world, and the Universe.[5]**

—Hyemeyohsts Storm, SEVEN ARROWS

\*   \*   \*

Preventive, ecological, medical ideologies are spreading partly because of a general recognition that many of the "controls" human beings have developed over nature have produced dangerous side effects. The speed with which scientific medical discoveries refute one another and the frequent ineffectiveness of modern medical techniques have made it clear to physician and client alike that no one system is omniscient. Everyone involved in the health professions is now encouraged to acknowledge the limits of their particular techniques and to allow for the participation of the patient, the possibility of new discoveries, and the chance of spontaneous cure. Regardless of symptoms and technical systems, the power of the individual will is being reasserted as the critical healing factor.

These attitudes are bringing preventive medicine back to its appropriate place within the system of the healing professions. The re-emphasis on patient participation in medicine and on self-healing makes our health care easier and less costly for the individual; it also requires more of an effort. We have gained more control over our own health along with more responsibility.

# A Preventive Approach to Health

**Apathy toward the work of wellness is a precursor of disease.**[6]
—Cythia H. Oelbaum, *American Journal of Nursing*

**One has the health that one works for.**[7]
—Hephzibah Menuhin, INTERVIEW WITH THE MUSE

A basic premise of preventive medicine is that it is more beneficial to ward off development of a physical problem than to have to cure yourself of it. Daily exercise, good diet and stress reduction are essential ingredients of any preventive health plan. Beyond the practical difficulties which may discourage one from regular exercise, one thing to bear in mind is that physical activity is not ultimately a spectator sport. Reflecting on it from afar has little to do with doing it. You'll never know its pros and cons until you feel it yourself, and your preventive program develops through experimenting with various movements and routines.

It is the nature of physical experience to take place in the realm of our metabolisms beyond the limits of the cerebral mind. This is why it is sometimes so difficult to move into the physical arenas when we are embroiled in mental tasks. This is also why we need free movement so much. It is a space in which we allow new responses to occur spontaneously. It is play; and play is a release from the pressure and monotony of mental work. Balancing work and play is vital to top capacity performance. Each activity refreshes us so that we may return to the other more fully.

As we attempt to keep our daily lives balanced we run into obstacles. Our culture is not built on the premise that preventive maintenance of our physical health is necessary. Almost all of us feel that time is a limited commodity. Corporations do not build gyms on the top floor for workers' exercise breaks. Even people who have physical jobs rarely have preventive health routines built into their work. And those of us who have the freedom to make our own schedules may feel guilty about taking time out from regular tasks to just move and enjoy it. Women especially must contend with their socially-programmed fears and ignorance of sports and exercise. Integrating regular exercise into our lives can bring about a change in self-image and requires faith in our bodies' ability to self-heal.

We all need to beware of the attitude that we might as well wait and see whether a mild physical problem becomes severe before bothering to attend to it. This outlook has led to countless bad backs, which could have been avoided by getting some exercise.

**What wouldst thou have, a serpent sting thee twice?**
—William Shakespeare, The Merchant Of Venice

## Getting Motivated

Sooner or later at some point, each of us feels a need to do more exercise. A brush with disaster may frighten some people into beginning preventive programs by impressing on them how precious their physical health is to all their functioning. Some people happen into the realm of the body by way of an interest in physically centered philosophies such as yoga. For others, the subtle changes the aging process brings about in the body are the motivation for beginning to exercise. We find that the older we get, the more we need to augment our bodies' automatic maintenance processes in order to stay in good health.

Whatever our initial motivation, we soon learn that keeping ourselves in top shape has some enticing aspects. We look better. We feel better physically and emotionally. Our medical bills decrease as our self-health programs become our doctors. We develop a fundamental strength which makes all our activities easier.

There is also the euphoria which comes from advanced physical activity. You hear of the "high" surfers experience riding the big wave, of the ecstasy found mid-air by ski jumpers, or of the pure joy experienced by a professional skater while making one more spin on the ice than she did the day before. You can experience moments of balance like these even in simple daily exercises. There is an irrepressible pleasure in doing a movement well for the first time or doing it with new-found ease. This increasing pleasure quota in your exercise is a key to getting hooked. That backbend you couldn't even approximate last week has become comfortable and easy. You know it will feel even better next time because you've found that after just a week of simple exercises, your muscle tone has improved and you now enjoy movements which initially felt jerky and difficult. Because you can actually feel your progress and with it a little more pleasure each day, you may begin to look forward to tomorrow's pleasant surprises. The payoffs for exercise in terms of increased body tone and stamina also come surprisingly quickly. After you begin to move, each motion becomes easier than the one before. Exercise is a self-escalating experience: the more you do, the more you can and want to do. The process becomes easy, and then irresistible.

Besides active euphoria there are many other positive effects of daily exercise: better circulation, a calmer mind, better health, more resilience. In the long run these benefits of improved health will get you hooked on your routine also. In the beginning, however, you'll need to recognize the immediate pleasures of the small changes in your movement capacity which will lead you to the next morning's routine.

## Body Awareness

At all stages of exercising, from the simplest to the most difficult, focus your attention on the inner body sensations. Just lifting your leg in a comfortable motion can be extremely pleasant. Your body craves smooth motion and will reward you generously for it. Notice that your grace improves from one movement to the next. When you are doing three leg lifts, the second will be easier than the first and the third will be easier still. Focus on the subtle movements of the muscles involved in any motion. You can savor a lot of small pleasures in your body movements if you can pay attention. At the end of your half hour's exercise these small pleasures add up to a larger feeling of well being. Over weeks, this feeling will grow and your body's state of pleasure will become deeper and longer lasting.

One of the reasons yoga is often more rewarding than many kinds of Western exercise is that it incorporates the principle of sensitivity. Yoga postures are distinguished from other exercise by the element of inner body attention the yogini is supposed to apply during each movement. This inner attention is a form of meditation which leads to a state of emotional peace. A lack of inner awareness is perhaps the reason that non-yogic exercise is often experienced as boring. However, you can apply your attention to the subtle body states you experience doing any exercises and increase the pleasure you derive from them.

Another aspect of yoga which we can learn to apply to any movement is the instruction not to push or strain, to go only as far as you feel comfortable. If you follow this suggestion you will notice that your body's range of movement will improve without stress. By simply doing the exercise as well as you're presently able you improve your physical state so that next time you will be able to do the exercise more easily. The amount of improvement that comes without pushing is a surprise to most beginners. It helps us understand the powers of non-aggression promoted by yoga. This gentle approach to exercise is also the best way to assure that you don't strain a muscle, twist a joint, pinch a nerve or otherwise hurt yourself while moving.

When you are ready to start exercising, compose your particular exercise routine from movements for each body part which feel best to you. If you feel a health problem coming on, start self-treatment of exercise, breathing, good diet and relaxation immediately before the problem has a chance to become severe.

# Getting Hooked on Feeling Good

Man prompted by his conscience, will through long habit acquire such perfect self-command, that his desires and passions will at last yield instantly and without a struggle to his social sympathies and instincts.
—Charles Darwin, THE DESCENT OF MAN

Most of us believe in exercise more than we practice it. How then do we get from the chaise longues to the squash courts? As I began writing about exercise and our resistance to it, most of the factors involved in a person's motivation toward health seemed clear. Yet I kept returning to one question: if we rational beings know that we'll feel, look and function better when we exercise, why do we hesitate? Boring as an exercise routine may seem to be, the minimal movement needed for good health is rarely gruelling or torturous. And the rewards for even the simplest exercise program are great. Why many people found regular exercise so difficult puzzled me.

After discarding the idea of using gimmicks or methods to trick yourself into healthful behavior I decided to look to some sages for understanding of this paradox. St. Thomas Aquinas, in "What Moves the Will?" of his SUMMA THEOLOGICA, circa 1267, says:

The intellect flies ahead, the desire follows sluggishly or not at all; we know what is good, but deeds delight us not.

Brilliant novelists like Virginia Woolf seemed to agree with this perplexity:

Why do I feel that there are severances and oppositions in the mind, as there are strains from obvious causes on the body? What does one mean by 'the unity of the mind,' . . . The mind is certainly a very mysterious organ.[8]

Turning from philosophy and art to science, I found a medical doctor, Leon Root, author of OH, MY ACHING BACK, who made an encouraging observation: "Those people who overcome their natural antipathy to exercise soon become devoted converts."[9] Still, this state comes *after* one has conquered resistance. What about the process of *doing* it?

Finally I found a simple passage from a book called WOMEN'S RUNNING by Dr. Jane Ullyot, which supplied a missing link in my logic and even made me feel like jogging. Dr. Ullyot says, "I run because I like to."[10]

Of course. You can force yourself to do things you don't like for short periods. But in the long run, we return to what we love, to what we think feeds us, to what we enjoy. The key to the mystery of motivation is pleasure. You have to find the exercise you like to do. Fortunately there are so many possibilities that there is truly an exercise for every taste. And if you like it—not just its results—you'll keep doing it again and again. You'll jog in Central Park at dawn, enter a skating rink in August, go around the block on your pogo stick, or attend tap dance class during lunch hour. You'll do it even if your family and the neighbors think you're nuts. You'll do it in the rain, sun, sleet, and snow. Because when you like doing it there are no problems with motivating yourself, no complicated philosophical arguments or appointments with the hypnotist. This secret of successful habit forming means that our quest is not to find the statistically healthiest activity but to find one we love to do, then allow ourselves to enjoy it.

Joy is healing. This is my philosophy. It's simple to understand and believe although somewhat more difficult to live. In my experience, a person heals through pleasure. This is the essence of miracle healing through love. When I say pleasure, I'm not referring to egocentric hedonism, but to balanced appreciation of all our capacities. In a practical daily context this means you gain most from non-stress stimulation and from movement which feels good. Body energy triggered by pleasurable experiences improves your whole state of being. We usually look and feel best when we are happy and often get sick when we are troubled.

There are endless types of exercise to choose from or create. Experiment with several kinds. Develop the ones which excite and please you. Don't push your body into painful states for the sake of competition. Be sensitive to your specific physical preferences and create a routine which is tailor-made for your body pleasures.

# Habit Forming

**Whenever I get the urge to exercise, I lie down until it passes.**
—Dr. Robert M. Hutchins, Former President of the University of Chicago

The following suggestions may help you take the steps to establish a regular health exercise routine in your life:

1. *Consider your attitude toward daily exercise.* If you discover that you think of your exercise period as a loss of time or energy, try to revise this outlook. Focus on exercise as profit. Think of what you gain: better health, good muscle tone, a better physique, improved circulation and a more relaxed attitude toward life. Exercise is also a reassertion of the positive parts of your natural animal state. Since many of us don't move much in our jobs or recreation, we need to exercise to maintain our agility and to stay in touch with the natural joy of movement.

2. *Make a place in your life for fitness;* create a special corner or set aside a separate room in your home for your exercise. Enter the space each day knowing you have succeeded in carving out a comfortable area in your life in which to maintain your health. Paint the room a relaxing color. Furnish it with comfortable firm mats, a zafu meditation pillow, some plants to help clean the air, and whatever gear you like to exercise with. Back balls, Ma Rollers, massage oil, barbells, towels, and good music can all be put to use. Ideally you should have enough clear space in which to lie down flat, to kick your legs wide, to jump rope high, to move freely. Wear appealing comfortable exercise clothes. In warm weather try exercising nude so you can move without restraint.

3. *Music* may inhibit and interfere with your own rhythm, or it may get you moving when nothing else inspires you. Experiment.

4. *Try public spas* and gyms to see if going to these facilities helps you exercise. You may be able to keep to a routine more easily if you are not working out at home. You may

find exercising with other people spurs you on. Invite a friend to join you at home or if you find the regularity of a daily or weekly class helpful, join a group.

5. *Approach the exercise in stages.* Don't set absolute goals for yourself such as establishing "a perfect new routine to last the rest of my life." This ambitious task may overwhelm and discourage you. Begin monthly or weekly projects to reach attainable goals. You might start by planning to do ten minutes of back exercises when you wake up. Next add ten minutes relaxation and stretching before bedtime. Then add a midday exercise break at the office. You can lengthen and embellish each period as you progress.

6. Be sure to *vary your routine* to keep your interest.

7. *Keep a role model in mind* while you are developing your routine. Changing our patterns involves changing our self-images. Pick someone especially inspiring as a model image for your routine. I like to remember that Greta Garbo is said to exercise each day and to especially love long walks. You may like to think of Willie Nelson as a jogger, Suzy Chaffee as a skier, Nureyev as a dancer, Esther Williams as a swimmer, Einstein as a cyclist, or Fred Astaire as a tap dancer. You may want to put their photos up in your exercise room next to your favorite picture of yourself at your healthiest. Finding out what your idols do to maintain their health may inspire you at a deeper level to stay in good shape.

8. Remember that one of the potential results of developing good exercise habits is the opportunity to *live your whole life at your fullest capacity.* When you are in good health all aspects of your life are enhanced and go more smoothly; you have a reservoir of strength to draw on when you deal with problems.

9. *Focus on your progress.* Take before and after photos. Note when you can touch your toes easily for the first time. Think of the svelte clothes you can wear when in good shape. Note when a formerly difficult backbend becomes easy. Note your decreasing medical bills and increasing stamina.

10. *Find the appropriate kind of exercise you love to do.*

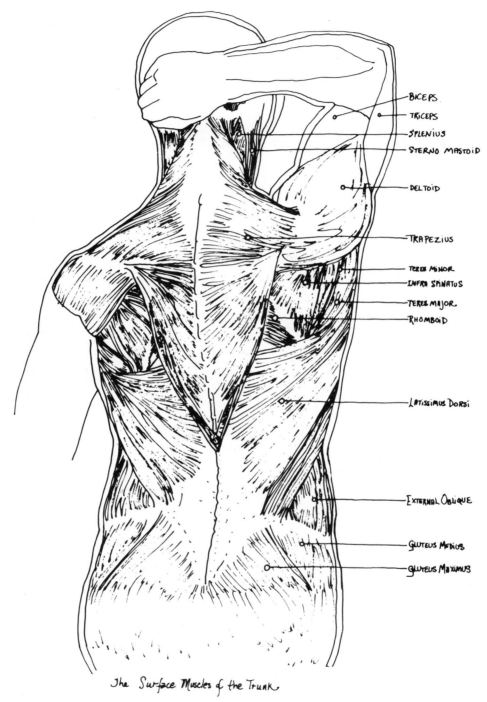

BICEPS

TRICEPS

SPLENIUS

STERNO MASTOID

DELTOID

TRAPEZIUS

TERES MINOR

INFRA SPINATUS

TERES MAJOR

RHOMBOID

LATISSIMUS DORSI

EXTERNAL OBLIQUE

GLUTEUS MEDIUS

GLUTEUS MAXIMUS

The Surface Muscles of the Trunk

# Anatomy
## Stephanie Mills

Stephanie Mills is a writer and editor whose primary concern is environment. She served as editor-in-chief of NOT MAN APART and EARTH TIMES magazines, and as associate editor of EARTH magazine. With Robert Theobald, she edited THE FAILURE OF SUCCESS, an anthology of readings on ecology and economics; and she edited and wrote an introduction to THE POPULATION ACTIVIST'S HANDBOOK. Her writing has appeared in THE WHOLE EARTH CATALOG, THE REALIST, CLEAR CREEK, THE COEVOLUTION QUARTERLY, PLAYGIRL, THE PACIFIC SUN, THE SAN FRANCISCO BAY GUARDIAN, and THE SAN FRANCISCO CHRONICLE. She has received foundation support for her salon, served on the boards of several organizations, and is currently working on a conference on technology. She has lousy posture and smokes, but swims about a half mile a day, and so far, her back feels just fine.

Understanding the workings of your spine and its musculature helps you understand some of what's happening as you exercise. The back, like every other part of the human body, is astoundingly complex. It's a curved stack of thirty-three bones—the vertebrae—which encircle the body's major nerve pathway, and are variously held upright and flexed by scores of different muscles. It's a fantastic and, as one writer put it, *audacious* piece of design; one which no amount of human imagining could have achieved.

In our possession of a spine, we are kin with all the living vertebrates—jawless fishes, sharks, frogs, snakes, woodpeckers, rats and a million other. Evolutionarily speaking, the spinal cord and backbone are the creatures' choice. A spinal cord is a mark of biological sophistication—it means that an animal's body is elaborate enough to require a routing system for nervous impulses travelling between the various organs and extremities and the brain.

The fact that back problems plague *homo sapiens* indicates the incompleteness of our audacious spine's evolution. We aren't ideally constructed for standing upright, and our inadequately built backs are constantly engaged in a struggle with gravity. Nevertheless, our structural adaptation is ingenious, and given a few million more years, may be more so.

## The Vertebrae

Nature's "engineering" is elegant: for instance, our vertebrae aren't in a straight stack. Instead, there are three curves in our spines—the cervical curve, in the region of the neck; the thoracic curve, in the region of the rib cage; and the lumbar curve at the lower back. The slight offsetting of each vertebra this series of curves achieves helps diffuse the force of compression. In the case of the lumbar curve, it also serves to bring our center of gravity over our legs, and transmits that force downward through the hip bones, which are among the strongest joints in the body.

Each vertebra forms a joint with the one below it, and although the range of movement between individual vertebrae is small, the range of flexibility in the spine as a whole is considerable, as anyone who has witnessed a yogi touch head to knees will agree.

Cushioning and limiting the movements of each vertebral joint are the notorious discs—capsules of connective tissue surrounding a gelatinous center. The discs are dandy little shock absorbers, but sometimes, under stress, the connective tissue gives way, and the nucleus pops out and presses against the spinal nerves. This painful occurence is known as slipping a disc.

There is a lot of variation in the form of the vertebra. Taking it from the top, our first vertebra is the atlas, so called after the Titan of classic mythology who bore the world on his shoulders. In us, the atlas merely supports the skull and its contents, a world of trouble perhaps, but not unbearable. The atlas is a wide open ring of bone, and not as spiny looking as the vertebrae below it; it interlocks with the second cervical vertebra, the axis, which has at the top a tooth-like projection on which the atlas pivots. The remaining five cervical vertebrae aren't quite so structurally specialized. What is most remarkable about our seven cervical vertebrae is their number, which is constant in every mammal, from humans to giraffes to whales.

The upper vertebrae are cylindrical, to accomodate the spinal cord, and have several bony projections radiating from their outer surfaces. One of these projections, or processes, serves to link each vertebra to the next. The others serve as points of attachment for that fantastic array of muscles which composes our back.

In the next group of vertebrae—the twelve thoracic vertebrae, some of these processes connect with our ribs, forming the joints which allow our chests to expand as we breathe. Moving on down the line, we come to the five lumbar vertebrae of our lower back, which, if the muscles surrounding them are weak, can suffer mightily under the load of our body weight. The spinal cord, as such, only runs as far as the lumbar vertebrae and becomes a tiny fibre as it enters the next five vertebrae which are the sacrum, the back wall of the pelvis. When we are born, the bones of the sacrum are separate, held

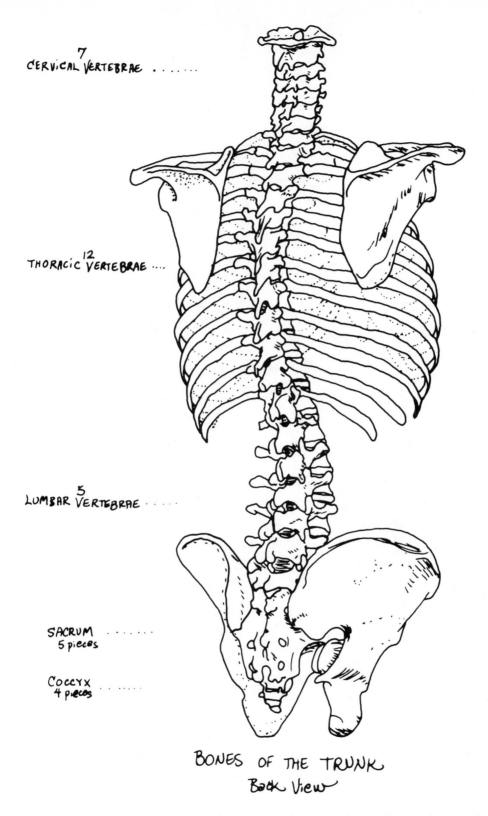

CERVICAL VERTEBRAE · · · · · · 7

THORACIC VERTEBRAE · · · 12

LUMBAR VERTEBRAE · · · · · 5

SACRUM · · · · · · ·
5 pieces

COCCYX · · · · · ·
4 pieces

BONES OF THE TRUNK
Back View

In man, the os coccyx, together with certain other vertebrae, though functionless as a tail, plainly represent this part in other vertebrate animals.

Charles Darwin, DESCENT OF MAN. 1871

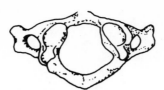

ATLAS: 1st CERVICAL VERTEBRA

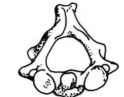

AXIS: 2nd CERVICAL VERTEBRA

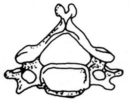

4th CERVICAL VERTEBRA

Upper View　　　　　Left Side View

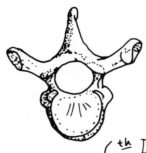

6th DORSAL VERTEBRA

Upper View　　　　　Left Side View

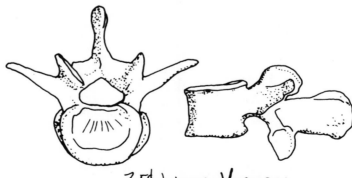

3rd LUMBAR VERTEBRA

Upper View　　　　　Left Side View

together by connective tissues. As we age, calcium phosphate, which rigidifies our bones, is deposited in the spaces between the sacral vertebrae, and usually by our twentieth year, unites these vertebrae as a solid mass.

At the bottom of the spine are the five coccygeal vertebrae which make the coccyx, or vestige of a tail. (Perhaps the anatomist who named the coccyx for its slight resemblance to a cuckoo's bill was too proud to consider that homo sapiens was not so far removed from other tail-wagging creatures.) The bones of the coccyx, separate when we are born, also grow together, and are usually joined by the time we reach thirty.

## The Muscles

Attached to all these vertebrae, and to our other bones, are groups of muscles. There are more than eighty muscles in and around the back. These may be roughly divided into three groups. The twenty-three pairs of deep back muscles are postural—they help us to stay erect. Some of these are short, connecting single vertebrae. Others run halfway down the back from the skull. As depicted in anatomical drawings, this muscular core of the back is a very ropy place.

Over it is another layer of a dozen pairs of muscles. Among these are the erector spinae, long thick muscles which run from the thoracic vertebrae to the sacrum. They're tough—you can feel them behind and under your ribs. Another of these paired muscles is the obliquus internus which stretches from a ligament in the pelvis up to the ribs. These muscles you can feel at your sides below your rib cage.

One of the biggest and most fundamental muscles of the back is the gluteus maximus, a pair of which make your bottom. This you should have no trouble finding. The gluteus maximus arises at the crest of the pelvis and connects with the upper leg bone, helping to pull us upright.

Among other sets of muscles in this middle layer are shoulder muscles. Over them, in the outer layer of the back's musculature are the trapezius muscles, two delta-shaped sheets running from midback and upper neck out to the shoulders. These help connect the arms to the spinal column, draw the shoulders toward the spine, and bend the neck to one side. There are plenty of other sets of muscles in the back, but an exhaustive description of them is beyond the scope of this chapter. (If you are interested in knowing more of what we are made of, lay hold of a copy of the current GRAY'S ANATOMY, Warwick & Williams, eds. W.B. Saunders Co., 1973. It's a staggering volume, describing us—our physical being—in minute detail.)

Tendons are the tough bands of connective tissue which unite our muscles with the bone and transmit muscular force. That force results from each muscle pulling just one direction. One of the reasons for the complexity of our musculature is that we need complementary sets of muscles, for pulling a bone or bones back and forth. When one muscle in a complementary set is working, the other is usually relaxed, except in isometric tension where both contract to hold one part of the body stationary so that another may

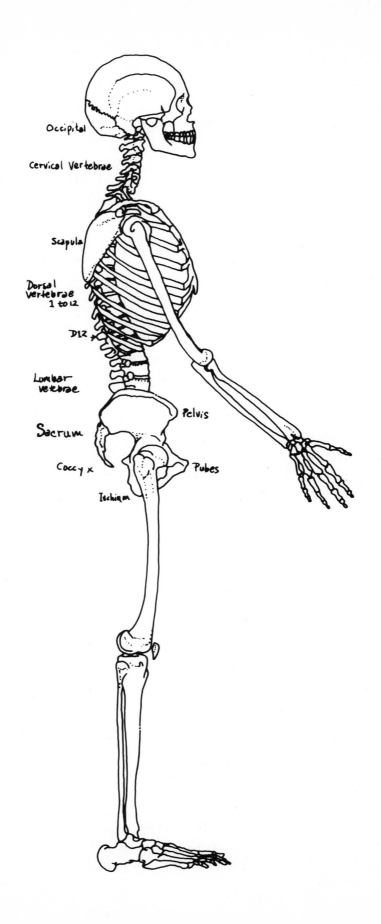

Occipital

Cervical Vertebrae

Scapula

Dorsal
Vertebrae
1 to 12

D12 ✗

Lumbar
vertebrae

Sacrum

Coccy ✗

Ischium

Pelvis

Pubes

move from it as a base. The striped muscle fibers which compose our skeletal muscles are bundles within bundles within bundles, which effect contractions within contractions at the signal of a nerve cell, or neuron.

## Blood Vessels

Muscle cells are nourished by extremely fine blood vessels called capillaries, whose walls are thin enough to bring the blood into contact with the cells. Capillaries are the farthest reach of the circulatory loop, diffusing oxygen-rich arterial blood to the cells and returning the blood by way of the veins to the heart and lungs to be recharged with oxygen again. Circulation also nourishes and purifies the blood as it runs through our different organs. This flow of blood fuels the muscle fibers, enabling them to contract in response to signals from the nerves. The long, threadlike nerve cells penetrate the bundles of muscle fiber and signal the need for movement, or to transmit sensory information back to the brain.

The spinal cord is the great conduit of these nerves. Thirty-one pairs of nerves run out from the sides of the spinal cord routing information to and from the voluntary muscles—those we can direct consciously—and to and from the smooth muscles of our organs, as well as relaying information from all our senses. With so much transmission and response going on all the time, the back begins to seem like a beehive of activity.

Our bodies contain worlds within worlds—and science only succeeds in revealing more infinity within. Given the time and space, we might describe the cells themselves, but perhaps this sketchy outline of one part of the human anatomy may tantalize you, and lead you to make that inquiry yourself—in between exercises, of course.

# II
# Prevention:
# If Your Spine is Fine

# Prevention—Section II: Contents

**Using This Book**

**A Basic Back Check**

**Moving Through the Day:** Waking Up; Neck Roll; Spine Line Up; Sitting to Standing; Standing; Walking; Back in the Office; To Sit; To Stand; Footstools; The Ideal Chair; Staying Alert; Rocking Chairs; The Chair Check-Up; Back in the Car; Driving; Rest Stops; Back on the Phone; Executive, Scholarly, and Musical Backs; Industry and Home Labor; Lifting; Back to Sleep

**A Physical Therapist: Marion Rosen**

**Warm Up: Flexibility Program:** Preparing; Marion Rosen's Exercises; Shoulder Jog; Stretch; Hitch Hike; Side Bender; Wing Rock; Hang Loose; Bend and Stretch; Hip Swing; Pelvic Rock; Knee Swing; Heel and Toe; Hip Circles; Rest; Knee Flops; Side Leg Lifts; Straight Leg Circles; Sit Ups; Final Rest

**Testing for Weak Points**

**Prevention Exercises:** Pelvic Tilt; Lower Back Leg Raise; Back Curl; Upper Back Opener; Salute to the Sun; Jump; Upper Back Release; The Fish; Arch; Neck and Spine Stretch; Head aches and Exercise; Holding Hands; The Squat; Hard Boiled Egg Rock; Sitting Up; Cracking Your Back; Resting

**Back to Back: Exercises for Couples and Groups**

**Emotions and the Back**

**A Therapist: Magdalene Proskauer**

**Visualization**

# Using This Book

To make the best use of the information in this book, keep the following pointers in mind as you exercise:

1. *Start slowly.* Gradually work your physical condition up to the point where you can perform the strenuous versions of the exercises. A gentle progress avoids muscle strain and gives your body time to develop the physical stamina which will make the exercises a pleasure rather than an ordeal.

2. *Choose exercises you enjoy.* There are many different kinds of exercises for different body parts and physical conditions. Find the ones you like which suit your particular style and rhythms.

3. *There's no gospel on the sequence of the exercises.* Do them in any order you like. The only wise rule to follow is to alternate a backward arch of the spine with a forward one. This keeps your muscles in balance and prevents cramps which result from emphasis on one kind of movement without its complement. If you get a cramp from arching your back too much, one of the best antidotes is to lie on the floor in a fetal position with your spine curled forward and to rest there awhile. Relax your muscles and imagine your breath moving freely up and down your spine.

4. Later in this section, there are several exercises called "Tests for Weak Spots." You may want to use these to *select the areas to focus on* as you exercise to rebalance your strength.

5. *Return every now and then to exercises that first seemed uncomfortable* and see whether your new flexibility makes those formerly unappealing ones enjoyable. Your range of body pleasure will increase as your tone and physical relaxation improve.

6. *Keep track of your changes.* If you record your progress in a Body Life Diary, you'll probably be pleasantly surprised at the extent and speed of your change. Without a record we often forget how we used to feel and how it felt to make the changes. This kind

of notebook can be of special use to teachers who guide students through cycles of progress.

7. *Don't do anything during exercise that hurts.* Don't accept professional treatments that are extremely painful. Any progress resulting from painful treatments will be temporary and your body will react and regress. Don't strain or push yourself during exercise. That isn't necessary for progress. Pain is a warning that your body is not ready for the movement. Listen to the messages and respect them. Otherwise, as Dr. Pat Grosh says, "Exercise is often a prime way to ruin your health."

8. *Always move smoothly.* Don't make sudden or jerky movements which might pull a muscle or joint. Flowing, gentle movement is the most healing to your body. Even high jumps and fast kicks can be done with ease, rather than stress.

9. *Synchronize your breathing and movement.* Inhale as you curl up; exhale as you stretch out. Don't hold your breath as you exercise. Try imagining your breathing as the force which lifts your limbs and relaxes your muscles. This helps improve circulation in the areas you are exercising, and steadies your movements.

10. *Your approach to exercising should, ideally, be noncompetitive.* That means not competing with what others may be doing, and not competing with yourself; not trying to stretch in uncomfortable ways, not trying to push your body too hard. You'll find that if you simply approximate each position according to what's comfortable for you, the next time you try it, you'll be able to do it better.

11. *Notice where the professionals interviewed in this book agree and disagree.* Their disagreements provide an important variety of perspectives. Their agreements, however, are even more interesting. I was impressed that in spite of their diverse backgrounds, each person agreed that preventive care and exercise make up the ideal back program. Each expert recommended drugs and surgery only in extreme emergency. Each stated he or she goes to other experts outside his or her specialty if necessary for treatment. This pragmatic openness is the basis for a sound holistic approach to medicine. I see the health approaches of the people interviewed as complementary, rather than exclusive. You can combine the energy and nerve treatments in acupuncture with the bone and muscle alignment of orthopedics to balance each. We can eliminate the need for one impossible system boasting all the answers by selecting the strengths of many systems.

12. *Adopt the exercises to your personal body condition.* If you have an injury which limits the use of your arms or neck, you can exercise other body parts to improve your muscle tone and general circulation. Or if you are handicapped by a paralysis in your lower limbs, for instance, you can still strengthen your back and shoulders by performing comfortable exercises lying down or sitting. Consult a variety of doctors and health professionals for their opinions if you have any problems.

13. *Don't repeat one movement too often.* Doing an exercise three or four times is plenty if you have been injured or strained. Too much repetition of a movement is often harmful because it can produce stiffness and pain. Proper breathing helps counteract

stiffness.

14. *Always include warm-up as well as cool-down periods in your exercise.* This entails starting slowly and increasing your exertion and pace gradually. Do stretching and limbering exercises first. The middle of your exercise period should encompass any strenuous activities. Alternate movement with rest and relaxed breathing. Then begin the cool-down phase: after peak exertion gradually decrease the pace of your exercises until you ease yourself into relaxation. Finally, lie down on the floor, close your eyes, and rest.

15. *While you're focusing on relaxing one body part, be sure you're not clenching another.*

16. *See if you can allow yourself to forget your life's other responsibilities and activities during your exercise period.* This will increase the benefits of your exercise by providing an emotional vacation from other pressures. The exercise period should be a time set aside just for you.

17. *As you do an exercise, ask yourself, "During which daily activity do I make this movement?"* The ultimate object of the exercises is to teach you to move through all your activities in a revitalizing way and to help you develop an everyday posture for pleasurable functioning.

# A Basic Back Check

I have a friend who is forty-seven, smokes, drinks lots of strong coffee, lives on Sixth Avenue in New York, spends much of her day curled over her writing desk, and refuses, principled woman that she is, to step into a hot tub. She is also distinguished by the fact that she has never had a back problem. Recently she presented this series of facts to me along with the challenging question of why the backs of health fanatics of all ages go out regularly, while she walks on upright.

After an investigation of the circumstances of her routines worthy of Sherlock Holmes, I unearthed the following explanatory factors: She has always insisted on sleeping on firm, flat beds. And when she was quite young she saw a sixty year old ballet star whose superb performance had an indelible impact on my friend's life. Her conclusion from seeing how beautiful the dancer looked and how gracefully she moved was that people who exercised enjoyed the benefits of radiance and agility late into their lives. She has exercised regularly since. These two life factors make her a model of back health despite her avoidance of hot tubs.

Our conversation prompted me to put together the following simple list of basic back health factors. The elements of good self health care are really very simple and are available to anyone. You can complicate the process according to your taste by surrounding the practices with a variety of healing philosophies. But in between theoretical questions, return to these functional ones and you should maintain a healthy spine.

If you are in good physical health and haven't had any serious accidents lately, but you feel a back ache condition coming on, you may want to run through the checklist in an attempt to pin down the cause of your new aches and pains. If you isolate the culprit(s) and change your approach to them accordingly, you can prevent minor discomfort from blossoming into a major problem. Refer to the chapters on these topics elsewhere in this book for more detailed information on the best way to cover each point mentioned for optimum care of your back. If you pass the self-exam, and your back ache persists, go see your medical doctor or health professional to check for internal or systemic causes of your problem.

| | |
|---|---|
| Exercise: | do you move well and get some limbering exercise each day? |
| Sleep: | do you sleep on a flat, firm mattress and use little or no pillow? Do you get enough sleep? |
| Posture: | is your functioning posture in good alignment? |
| Shoes: | do you wear low-heeled shoes, in a comfortable size, with thick enough soles to cushion your step? |
| Chairs: | do you spend much working time sitting, in stiff positions? |
| Car: | do you drive a lot; does your car have a comfortable driver's seat? |
| Posture Breaks: | do you take breaks during the day to release body tension? |
| Accidents: | have you had any major or minor falls or twists lately? |
| Stress: | is some element in your life causing you excess emotional stress and tension? |
| Change: | have you made any significant changes lately, bad or good, to which you may be reacting? |

**If you're into backs, take care of the one you've got.**
—Bill Graham

# Moving Through the Day

### Waking Up

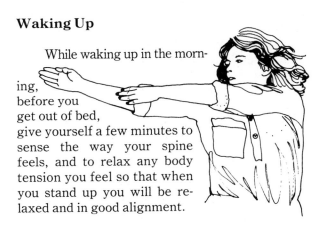

While waking up in the morning,
before you
get out of bed,
give yourself a few minutes to
sense the way your spine
feels, and to relax any body
tension you feel so that when
you stand up you will be relaxed and in good alignment.

### Neck Roll

If you wake up lying on your stomach, roll over onto your back, bend your knees, and align your head, spine and hips in a straight line. In this position, roll your head gently from side to side to relax your neck. Be sure that you breathe comfortably. Now gradually begin to roll your arms so that as you roll your head to the left, both arms also roll over to the left. As you roll your head to the right, bring your arms across your chest and over to your right side. Create a gentle swaying motion with your head and your arms moving together. Inhale as you raise your arms and exhale as you lower them. This helps relax any tightness between your shoulder blades and along your neck, which might result from sleeping on your stomach or sleeping with your neck in a strained position.

### Spine Line Up

This exercise is basic to spinal alignment. It is repeated throughout the book because it is good for you at any stage. Relax your arms at your sides; bring your head to the center. Inhale as you push down with your feet and lift your pelvis off the bed. Slowly lift the rest of your spine up to your shoulder blades off the bed. Let your spine hang unstrained awhile, as though suspended between your knees and shoulders. Now exhale while you lower your spine back onto the bed: release each vertebra, starting with the vertebrae between your shoulder blades first and progressively working your way down toward your sacrum and hips. Your hips should be the last part of your body to rest on the bed again. Do this lifting and releasing sequence several times.

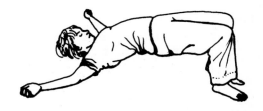

### Sitting To Standing

Prepare to get up out of bed by rolling over onto your side almost in a fetal position, with your knees bent and pulled toward your chest and your chin tucked under. Raise your body to a sitting position by pushing with your arms rather than straining with your neck and back. Then come to a standing position.

Good posture is not just keeping your body in correct alignment while you're still. Throughout the day, be aware of your active posture. All the exercises in this book are designed to develop your awareness of the most comfortable and flexible positions for your body during all kinds of movement.

### Standing

When you're standing, a good portion of your body weight should rest on your heels, and your chest should be slightly lifted and forward. Your knees should always be slightly flexed. Tuck your pelvis under so that your stomach is not protruding because this produces lower back strain.

Stand and walk with your toes pointed comfortably forward. Your feet are major supports for your body. Thus you want to maximize the area of that support by placing your feet at least as far apart as your shoulders, and pointing your toes forward so that you not only have a wide base reaching from side to side, but also from back to front. Be sure you're not tilting your feet to either side, thus straining your arches or your other foot muscles.

Prolonged standing is always a strain on your body and should be avoided. If your work requires you to stand for a long time, be sure to keep your knees flexed as you stand, and take frequent movement breaks, like bending your knees and squatting. If you can't squat where you work, bend your knees and lift your legs; shift your weight from one foot to the other; move your arms and shoulders; and keep reviewing your body posture to be sure that you're in good alignment. Move as much as you can while you're standing so that your weight is not compressed on one body area for a prolonged time.

Many people tend to shift their weight backward in an attempt to relax their muscles while standing. This should be avoided because it increases the pressure on your lower spine. Shifting your weight forward with bent knees decreases the pressure on your lower back.

Choose your shoes carefully. High heels increase the problem of weight pressing on your lower back by encouraging a curve in your lower spine, and increasing the pressure on the vertebrae near your waist.

If you have to stand for long periods you can also relieve the strain in your back by using a foot rest for one of your feet. This also helps prevent swayback. If you place one foot up on a small footstool, it helps to flatten the curve in your lower back and relieve some of the pressure in that area.

### Walking

When walking you should be sure to keep your chest uplifted so that it, rather than your abdomen, is the more forward part of your body. This and tucking your hips under help relieve pressure on your lower back and prevent you from immobilizing your lower back as you walk. Keeping your lower back stiff makes walking difficult and strains your back. Also be sure to lift your knees when you walk so that you're flexing your leg and lower back muscles. Don't walk with your knees straight because this forces you to strain your knees and throw your legs out to the side in order to move forward. As you lift your leg, your pelvis should tilt under and forward, and as you step down your pelvis should tilt up and back. This co-ordinated movement is important for maintaining flexibility of the spine.

Pay attention to your breathing as you walk. A good pattern is to inhale when you lift your leg and exhale as you put it down.

\* \* \*

**Exercise is what you do to get from your apartment to a taxi cab.**[11]
Fran Leibowitz, METROPOLITAN LIFE

\* \* \*

## Back In The Office

### To Sit

People often strain their necks and backs by lowering their hips into a chair while holding their necks upright. Sitting down in this position is uncomfortable for your back. When you're about to sit down, stand close to the chair. Set your feet almost under it, and bend your hip joints and knees. Tuck your chin under and incline your torso forward. This distributes your weight over your feet. Otherwise the strain will be on your back. As you bend your knees and lower your pelvis into the chair, your torso should be almost parallel to the floor. Thus the weight of your body will be lowered into the chair by your thighs, calves, and feet rather than by your back. Then when your pelvis is on the seat of the chair, lean your torso into an upright position.

### To Stand

To rise from the chair, simply reverse the motion described above. Rock your torso forward at the hips, keeping your spine straight and your chin tucked under toward your chest. Roll the weight of your body onto your feet as you lean forward. Keep your torso parallel to the floor until you can straighten your legs. The last thing to straighten is your spine. It's good to practice standing and sitting in a continuous motion so that you get used to this, rather than straining your back. Once you get into the habit of sitting and rising in this pattern, you'll find it becomes a pleasurable, rocking, circular motion.

### Footstools

To maintain good posture when you're sitting down, rest your feet flat on the floor and bend your hips and knees at approximate right

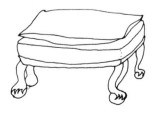

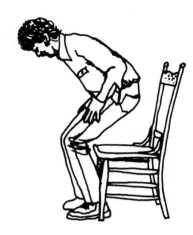

angles. Most people agree that having your knees a little higher than your hips is preferable. This can be achieved by either sitting in a chair low enough that your knees are slightly elevated or by using a small footstool to raise your knees above the level of your hips. This elevation will take the pressure off your lower spine, help you straighten out your lower back, and open up the areas in the back which sitting in the wrong position can compress.

### The Ideal Chair

Your chair should have forearm support so that your arms can rest on the arms of the chair at about elbow level. In this position your shoulders can relax without having to carry the weight of your arms. Be sure the arms of your office chair fit under your desk. When you're buying a chair keep all these requirements in mind, and try the chairs in the store. If you have chairs at home that need adjustment, you can make them more comfortable by putting cushions on the seat to make it higher, adding cushions to the back to help flatten your spine when you're sitting, or by using a footstool with chairs that are too high for your leg length. It's important also that the seat be deep enough to permit you to sit all the way back in the chair. Otherwise there will be pressure on your calves and the backs of your knees. If the chair is too deep, then put a firm cushion on the back of the chair. The idea is to maintain your posture as effortlessly as possible while you're sitting. Constantly tensing to hold your body in one position gives you muscle cramps.

\*    \*    \*

**Between man and nature stands culture.**[12]
—Alfred Grotjahn

\*    \*    \*

One good way to maintain your sitting balance with minimum effort is to broaden your base of support. Because your spine is only one small point, try to distribute your weight to your hips and your thighs so your base of support will be greater. If you don't have a footstool and your chair is too high, you can tuck your pelvis under and cross your legs to help relieve the pressure on your lower spine. You should alternate the crossed leg often though to avoid cramping the circulation in your legs.

While you're sitting down reading or just having a conversation with someone, shift your position every now and then so that your body doesn't get stiff. Check to be sure that your spine is in good alignment and that you haven't slumped. Higher-backed chairs provide good support for people with upper back or neck pains.

For sitting down at work, it's important that you have an adjustable chair that meets all the requirements for comfort. You should sit well back in the chair with your weight on your ischia, the lower back bones of your pelvis, and not on your spine. When you move forward to lean on the desk or to write, don't bend at the waist or in your chest. Bend at your hip joints. This prevents extra pressure on your vertebrae. Your arms should be supported by the desk or table in front of you at a comfortable level so that your spine isn't strained by the height of the table. To offset fatigue, shift the position of your body frequently while you're working.

**Staying Alert**

If you have a job which requires you to be at your desk for long periods of time, change sitting positions often; stand up and walk around the room frequently, and do some simple exercises to encourage your circulation. Do squatting positions so that your knees don't cramp. Get up and move around as often as you can.

There is an entire laboratory at New York University Medical Center, the Institute of Rehabilitation in Medicine, which is devoted to studying job efficiency as related to good health. There may be similar clinics in your area, and if you feel your company does not give enough consideration to its employees' occupational health, you might investigate programs to recommend to your industry or employer. You can point out that it's to your company's advantage for you to be healthy and comfortable while you're working because your productivity and the quality of your work will increase if you are.

If you feel that the chair that is provided for you at the office isn't right, see if you can get your company to buy you a new one. If not, it would probably save you a few doctor's bills to buy yourself a chair and bring it to the office. You want a chair that will support the structure of your body and will permit the kind of movement that you need to make while you're working. The chair is an extension of your skeleton in the sense that it holds up your body when you are working and moving. So it's very important that it be in the correct proportion to your body and have the right design for you to function well while in it.

Back pain usually is caused by nerve irritation resulting from the compression of ruptured vertebrae discs. Other common causes of back pain are arthritis, nerve disease, body asymmetry and scoliosis. You can usually prevent these common ailments by avoiding excess pressure on your vertebrae, compression of the spine, and pinched nerves.

If you have back trouble, ideally you should have a chair in which the erector muscles of the lower spine can be released from spasm and any local swelling reduced, while activity is still possible. You want to shift the upper body weight from the disc onto the chair back. The most obvious position for this is reclining, so you may need a reclining chair. To keep your back healthy, lie back in your chair from time to time and take a rest.

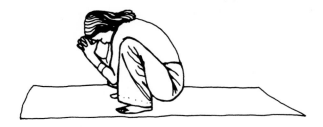

Squatting is a good resting position. This is really the perfect sitting posture, although in our culture it is socially unacceptable in most situations to squat. Elsewhere in the world many people do squat, however, and they usually have better spines than most executives. Since we are ordinarily confined to sitting on chairs, in order to relieve the pressure on your lower spine from time to time, you can go in the bathroom and squat, or squat by your desk if you have a private office.

## Rocking Chairs

Dr. Janet Travell, who was President Kennedy's personal physician, recommended he get a rocking chair to use in his White House office because old fashioned rockers are really a perfect chair for the back.

You can put your feet up on the front rungs of the chair; this helps elevate your knees higher than your hips. Rocking chairs usually have straight backs with openings at the lower part; and they have arm rests. Also the fact that you can rock in the chair prevents you from getting cramped into one position. The rocking movements of the chair also relieve your back of some of the work of standing and sitting. It would be ideal for you to have a rocking chair in your office to move to when you have to read, talk on the phone, or meet with people.

If you're an artist and work on a stool at a drafting desk, make sure that the stool has rungs on which you can rest your feet so that your knees are positioned slightly higher than your hips.

A typing table is usually between twenty-two and twenty-four inches high, usually a good height depending on how tall you are. For your comfort, be sure that your chair is the correct height in relation to your table so that you don't have to strain your arms and back to reach the typewriter. An adjustable chair seat is good for this purpose because you can change its height for different activities.

Chairs should provide some support for your back at your belt line, including the vertebrae between the top of your sacrum and the bottom of your ribs. This area needs a little extra support when you're sitting. People who sit down at work sometimes get sciatic nerve pain because their chairs are structured so that sitting compresses the spine and pinches the nerves. They also forget to move around and relieve the pressure on the spine that comes from sitting for long periods. Do your favorite breathing exercises at your desk to increase your circulation and oxygen intake. Every now and then lean forward in your chair and rest your head and torso on your thighs, with your arms relaxed toward the floor, to relieve lower back pressure from sitting. And as often as possible, remember to get up and move!

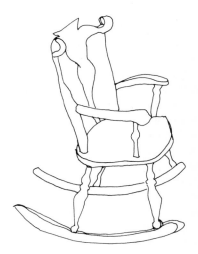

## Chair Check-Up

Dr. Travell suggests nine things to look out for in chairs:

1. Be sure that the chair supports your lower back. Lack of this support is probably the commonest flaw in store-bought furniture. If you spend hours in such a chair, your muscles become fatigued from having no lower back support. You can relieve this fatigue by putting a cushion in the back of the chair to help support your upper back without putting strain on your lower back.

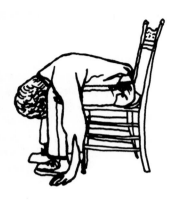

2. The chair may be too curved at shoulder level so that your upper back doesn't have any support. This may cause you to slump your shoulders forward and strain your upper back muscles.

3. If the arm rests are too high, they will push your shoulders forward, which strains your upper back.

4. If the back of the chair isn't sloped enough, but is perfectly straight, it's bad for your back because it may cause you to droop forward and develop round shoulders.

5. If the back of the chair is too short, which is often true in movie theatres, the result may be stress on your shoulders and neck.

6. Another problem is jack-knifing at the hips or at the knees. If your knees are too high, as they may be on a bar stool or in some cars, then you overstretch your back muscles and get cramps. This also happens in chairs with low seats and high front edges, so you can use a wedge-shaped cushion in the seat to raise the seat at the back and make it fairly horizontal.

7. During World War II many people came to doctors with swollen feet. These people had often been sleeping in air raid shelters on folding deck chairs. The pressure of the edge of the deck chairs against the back of the thighs just above the knees had cut off the circulation in their lower legs by pressing on the spot where the artery and veins cross the bones. Be sure that your chair doesn't do this, and don't sit in a deck chair for long stretches of time. Any chair with a high, hard front edge can produce this condition.

8. Bucket seats can also be a problem. They put the weight on the sides of the buttocks so that you sag in the center, and roll your thighs inward. The muscle distortion resulting from sitting in this position causes back discomfort and strain.

9. If the chair is the wrong size for you and you have to dangle your feet so the weight of your legs compresses the blood vessels under your thighs and shuts off some circulation, get a footstool. And be careful that your chair seat is not too deep. You should be supported by the back of the chair without having to sit so far back that the circulation in your legs is cut off.

## Back in the Car: Driving

The car seat should be far enough forward so that your knees are slightly higher than your hips. This reduces lumbar lordosis. The car seat should not be so far back that your knees are lower than your hips and your legs extended, so that you have to strain your back and leg muscles to reach the pedals. Car seats come in very different shapes. According to several doctors, Volvos, Saabs, Mercedes, Volkswagen Rabbits, Audis, and Cadillacs that have electric seats are kindest to your back.

You can change the shape of your car seat by using pillows. Sit on firm pillows to reduce the

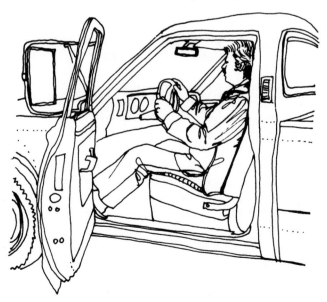

bucket shape of bucket seats, and use firm pillows to give your lower and middle back support. You may also want to put a cushion under your knees if the car seat tends to cut off the circulation in your lower legs.

### Rest Stops

When you stop to take a rest on the side of the road, walk around the car, stretch, and do several squats. If the seat reclines, lie down in your car to give your back a rest.

When driving for long periods of time, it's very important not to let your hip joints become cramped and pinched. So swing your knees from side to side occasionally as you're driving to relax your hip joints. Change your position and lean forward in your car seat every now and then so that your lower back doesn't get compressed.

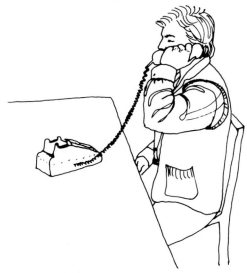

### Back on the Phone

If you are a secretary or an executive and have a job which requires you to talk on the phone a great deal, it's important to avoid neck and upper back cramps. Ideally, you would have the kind of phone which is like a small intercom, that sits on your desk and has no receiver at all. If you have a regular telephone, however, hold the phone to your ear without tilting your neck to one side. If you tilt your neck to the side while you're talking on the telephone for a long time, you may develop muscle cramps.

### Executive, Scholarly, and Musical Backs

Executives' lives have many back-traps. Most executives sit down a great deal of the time in meetings, or at their desks; and to maintain a healthy back it's important to get up and walk around and move the body to promote flexibility, improve circulation, and prevent cramps. Most executives travel in their cars a lot and this can be harmful because it means so such sitting down; in this position even more body weight is pressing on your spine than when you are standing.

Many people who sit down a great deal develop back problems (often sciatica) as well as an imbalance in the leg muscles and length. This phenomenon is often due to the long hours a person sits on a slightly tilted surface which presses on the sciatic nerve; this culprit is often a wallet in a truck driver's, a drummer's, or an executive's back pocket. If you sit down a lot, keep your wallet in your breast pocket or purse, and your happy back muscles will save you money.

Remember whenever you can, avoid sitting down; move around instead. When you travel in airplanes be sure to recline your seat, and to get up and walk around the plane whenever you can. Use those small pillows that are provided to improve the shape of the airplane seat, so that your lower back has support and you're not sunk in a bucket seat.

If you are a musician who sits for long periods or who plays an instrument with your arms held in the same position for extended time, you may develop back cramps. Do exercises for the sore areas in your back and try to vary your playing position to avoid cramps. Use footstools to offset back strain whether you play standing or sitting.

### Industry and Home Labor

If you work in a job where you lift heavy objects or even if you only lift something once a day, it's very important to have your body in the right position. Studies of industries in which workers do a lot of lifting have shown that lifting things safely depends on worker fitness, and a combination of environmental conditions, such as temperature, humidity, time of day, distance of the load from the body, configuration of the object to be lifted, frequency of lifts, worker position during the lift, and the starting point of the lift.

## Lifting

A labor study done at the Allis-Chalmers' Combine Division in Independence, Missouri, indicated that given perfect work conditions and fit workers, an employee could be expected to lift fifty pounds about four times a minute from floor to knuckle height; fifty pounds six times a minute from knuckle to shoulder height; and forty-five pounds six times a minute from shoulder to full overhead extension. There are many more standards that have been developed from this study done on lifting, so that there is now a table of statistics about what size worker is capable of lifting what weight box how many times a minute. If you are working in a factory you might want to read such labor studies for ideas on labor conditions and the amount of such work you can reasonably be expected to do.

You don't have to be working in a factory to strain your back while lifting. You can do it at home by lifting a box out of the closet, by carrying groceries from the car, by picking up a child, or by even picking up a pencil. It all depends on what shape you're in, how much stress you're under, and how well you move your body.

Any heavy lifting should be done with slight flexion of the hips and considerable flexion of the knees so that you lift mainly with the muscles in your thighs and legs, rather than with the muscles in your back. Also, keep your elbows slightly bent and your pelvis tucked under.

The best way to lift an object from the floor is to squat all the way down and pick up the package while squatting. Then stand up so that you use your leg muscles to do the lifting. Don't arch your back; keep the lumbar region straight when

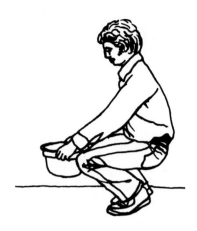

you squat and keep one foot flat on the floor at all times.

Here are some simple rules for work movement which will help you avoid back problems:

1. Avoid bending from the waist. Always bend at your hips and knees. Squat low to lift an object up. Never bend over without flexing your knees and tucking your buttocks under.

2. Avoid lifting heavy objects above waist height.

3. Face the object you wish to lift as you reach for it, rather than reaching sideways.

4. Avoid carrying unbalanced loads.

5. Always hold heavy objects close to your body.

6. Never carry or move anything so heavy or awkward that it causes you to strain.

7. Avoid sudden movements. Learn to move smoothly.

8. Change positions frequently. This keeps you from getting cramps and maintains your flexibility.

9. When you're mopping, vacuuming, raking, hauling, or doing any kind of work that requires you to bend over, work with the tool close to your body, and take relatively small

\* \* \*

**I helped plant (cotton); I hoed it, picked it, chopped it and hated every minute of it. I feel like Charley Pride feels. I don't ever want to walk through a cotton field again. Every time we pass one in the bus I get a back ache.**[13]

—Tammy Wynette

\* \* \*

steps. Don't reach too far from your body when you're sweeping or hauling. Just make reaches that are easily within the scope of your motion.

10. When you dress yourself, do it sitting down rather than straining your back by standing up and bending over.

11. Wear low-heeled shoes.

12. Avoid activities which arch or strain your lower back like extreme backward or forward bends.

13. When you cough or sneeze, round your back slightly and bend your knees.

14. When you are making the bed, or doing any work which requires bending or stretching, try doing it in a kneeling, rather than a standing position. Keep your pelvis tucked under as you stand up.

15. Remember to let your head and neck relax forward when you bend over, or stretch forward, rather than keeping your neck rigid, so that your neck isn't pulling in the opposite direction from your back. You should also remember to alternate any one kind of physical activity with some other motion, so that you don't get cramps from repeating the same motion over and over. Above all, don't let yourself get out of shape or too weak because in that condition you can easily strain your muscles.

## Back to Sleep

Sleep on a firm, flat mattress. Choose one that feels really comfortable. Too soft a surface may allow your spine to arch too much; too hard may make you ache, or pinch a nerve from too much pressure all night. Sleep on your back, or your side with your knees bent and a pillow between your knees. Lying on your stomach arches and strains the neck and lower back. Use only a small thin pillow or no pillow at all to keep your spine straight. If you must use a pillow, try one of the small cervical pillows. They support your neck slightly rather than tilting it enough to strain it. If you sleep on your back put a pillow under your knees and ankles for support. Sleep in a dark, quiet room, that's not overheated. Try keeping a diary of your dreams especially those containing body images. After several months read it consecutively as the story of your inner cycle.

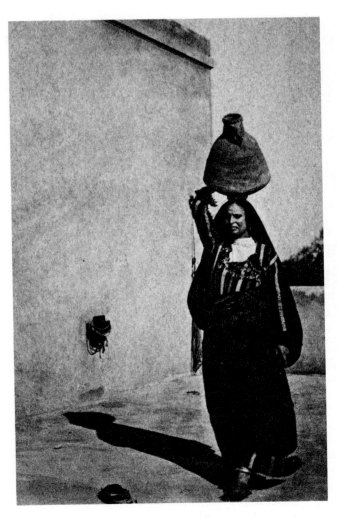

\* \* \*

The exercises in this chapter help you learn to move in ways so you avoid straining your back in your daily routine. The exercises in the following chapters should help you strengthen your muscles and increase your maximum capacity.

\* \* \*

Anne Kent Rush

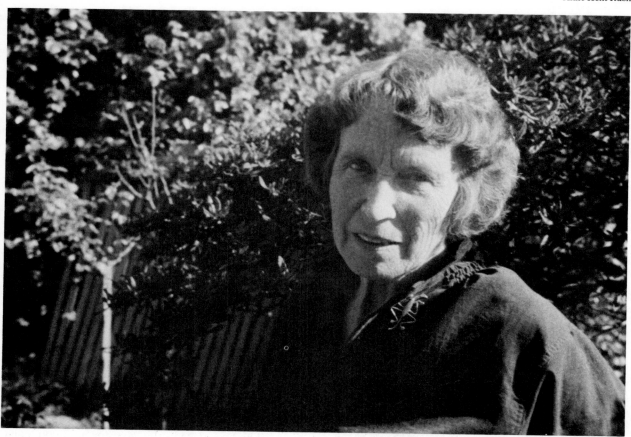

Marion Rosen

# A Physical Therapist: Marion Rosen

Marion Rosen began her training in Munich in 1936 with Dr. Gustav Heyer and his assistants, studying breath and relaxation techniques combined with psychotherapeutic treatment. In Sweden in 1939 she participated in a physical therapy training course and took her official exam in Stockholm. Rosen came to the U.S. in 1940 to take premedical studies at the University of California, Berkeley. In 1944, she attended the Mayo Clinic's training course in physical therapy and took the National Registry Exam. She worked as a Physical Therapist at Kaiser Hospital in Richmond, California until 1946, when she went into private practice. Recently Marion Rosen's work has become re-focused on relaxation techniques, because she "found this approach most effective in the long run." She is on the staff of the Psychosomatic Medicine Clinic in Berkeley and continues her private practice. Her current work concerns body awareness and her techniques combine massage, posture education, exercises for limbering body structure through joint flexibility, and breathing techniques. She teaches classes for men and women of all ages in several centers in Berkeley, and sees private patients in her office in Oakland.

## Posture and Mobility

Because I am a physical therapist, many people with acute back problems come to me. It is not very hard to treat an acute case. The real difficulties are in treating people who have chronic backaches. I have found that two factors are critical when you work with a person suffering from backache. One of these is to develop mobility of the musculature. The second is to develop good posture.

I define good posture as 'the way to carry your body with the least amount of effort.' Does the spine really balance itself? Actually it should need little support from the musculature. The muscles are there to move the bones of the spine, not to hold them. When we use back muscles for holding instead of moving, we get in trouble. I try to teach people how to move, how to use their musculature and how it feels to be aligned in the right way.

I find in most cases that if it is possible for a person to become properly aligned and to move well, then backaches are not a problem. In cases where people's backs are causing them pain, I would first show them simple remedial exercises to be done every day rather than the limbering exercises I teach my classes. There is a set of exercises called Williams' Flexion Exercises recommended by most orthopedic doctors for people who have back troubles. These are effective, simple and good. However, I would ask someone without an acute problem to do more maintenance exercises. People who usually just work one set of muscles in their professions need an additional set of exercises to keep their bodies in a good state of flexibility.

The way our bodies are made, we need to move every part at least once in twenty-four hours to retain our mobility. I have developed a series of exercises for the joints. I call it "joint hygiene," because you must move the joints to keep them at their maximum mobility potential. Most people move their whole body in the course of the day, unless they have a sedentary occupation, like psychiatry or office work, and they sit in one position hours at a time. These people really have to exercise in order to get their bodies working the way they should.

Because of its structure, the back is more apt to suffer from disuse and tension. So a lot of my therapy focus is on back movements. The back is structurally prone to problems because we don't walk on all fours any more. Since we walk upright, one area of the back, around the fourth and fifth lumbar vertebrae, is set at a particularly precarious angle. If that angle gets exaggerated in any way by posture or activity, back troubles often result. It is important that the pelvic and lower back relationship is at its best. If you lose the balance of the spine, you have to re-learn it.

Even if your back doesn't ache, you may not have enough movement in your life. It still could be necessary to do some exercises corresponding to the exercises I've developed which are actually a preventive physical therapy. I have always given these exercises to loosen up a person who has tight shoulders or hip joints, low back pain or any pain in the spine. I now give these same exercises to prevent people from getting stiff or losing their range of function.

The spine has many small joints, and every joint has to move to stay lubricated. The lubricating synovial fluid in the joints forms even if you just move the joint once a day. But if you do not move it, the joint runs dry.

Over the years I have worked with a lot of people with back problems. Often people with acute back problems have lifted something and hurt a small muscle fiber, or had something fall on their backs which caused a contusion. An injury such as this resulting from an accident, is likely to heal after rest. However, chronic back problems come from bad postural habits or disease. The treatment for chronic conditions is more difficult because it involves a subtle re-education of habit patterns. When someone comes to me with chronic back pain, I first look to see where their tensions are. When they have a low back pain the low back is not necessarily the culprit. Very often the tension originates in other parts of the body. So it wouldn't help to only give them low back exercises. The therapist must see that the rest of the body is flexible. Because the whole spine works as one, a person cannot take on good posture in the low back unless the upper back follows suit.

Sometimes I will prescribe a special set of exercises for people, and they recover from their problems. But they may come back five years later and say, "I have back pains again." I ask them, "Did you do the exercises?" They say, "I did them for three years and stopped. Then the pain came back." As long as they kept the spine moving, they could function without pain. Thus mobilization seems to be the most important factor in preventive care.

A second important factor is posture. But you cannot have good posture unless you also have mobility of the spine. To explain visually what the correct posture is, I have the person stand in front of a mirror and I show them the difference between one posture and the other. They can both feel and see where their weight shifts. For instance, when you push your pelvis backward you can see that your stomach hangs out in front and the shoulders hang incorrectly. The moment the pelvis is tucked under the rest of the body, everything changes: the shoulders and the back become straighter; the stomach is held in the pelvis; the upper back straightens up without effort because the back is held up by the bones of the spine and pelvis.

I also call attention to the improvement in their looks. They can see for themselves how much better they look when their bodies are aligned than when they're not. Next, I talk about anatomical structure. Then I focus on how you feel when you hold your body up without effort or stress. You can feel your bones holding you up, so you can relax your muscles. Then I show them movements to practice to learn how to function in this good alignment without effort.

The sound you hear when someone "cracks" your back is a vacuum pop that may happen in places that haven't been moved for awhile. The little twisting movement opens a space between the spinal vertebrae, causing the synovial fluid to form again so that the joint gets lubricated. So back cracking is an important aspect of back hygiene. In Java and some other Oriental countries, school children are taught how to move, how to crack their necks, how to crack their spines, and how to make sure that their joints are totally movable and lubricated. This is very wise because what people have to do to stay healthy is move. There's no other way. This is why modern sedentary life is so hard on our bodies.

If you are ill and having physical therapy, you do not necessarily have to move your limbs yourself nor do you have to move strenuously. Physical therapists are often asked to move the patient's joints. This helps avoid stiffening of the joints. Each joint has a definite set of movements and a range of motion. Whatever movements a particular joint allows you must make, in order to keep it supple. You can invent your own exercises if you know what a joint's possibilities are. Some joints, like the knee, just bend and stretch.

Other joints, like those in the hips and the shoulders are ball-and-socket joints which can roll all the way around. There are many joints in the foot that move as you step. You have to do all kinds of little movements in order to move the joints sideways and up and down.

## The Neck

The place where the neck goes into the shoulder at the cervical vertebrae is usually hard to move. It's an important part of the spine because it's a center of force and the junction of a group of muscles that go up to the head as well as down from the shoulders to the mid-back. That point must be flexible in order to permit free movement of the upper back and neck. This is the spot where people develop what's called "dowager's hump." Dowager's hump is often caused by bad posture. If you sag in your chest, your head will hang forward. Then because you can't see well in this position, you tend to tilt your head backward. To straighten out the neck you need to relax. So many of us have forgotten how to relax our necks. We can't merely stretch to relax our necks—we have to release muscle tension. Because there is nothing structural to pull the head up we just have to let the skull relax onto the spinal column for support. The Alexander Alignment Method has some fine exercises which teach you to relax and let your neck straighten up. This takes pressure off the base of the neck.

If people have no physical complaints, but can't get into an exercise routine, then I say, dance. The people who come to my exercise classes don't exercise during the week. They just move well. When you really move well as you go through the motions of simple chores, such as reaching for something, or vacuum cleaning, or whatever you do, if you really enjoy the movement fully, I do not think you need to exercise. Routine exercises are for people who don't have occasion to move much of their bodies in their way of life.

When I say to dance, it doesn't matter what kind. Just play music and be abandoned. Let go as you move. Really move your whole body. You can see from the way people look if what they do is good for them. Does your body seem to support its life and flexibility without stress? When you feel your neck getting stiff sitting at a desk, the neck is telling you you'd like to have some movement. If you listen to your body, it lets you know.

I think the key factor for health is the joy of living. Health is a body working at its best. There is a certain contentment which has to do with fulfillment. It doesn't matter whether you're a writer who sits all day at a desk, or a person who hikes in the mountains. As long as you love what you do, your fulfillment inside and out will be complete—and evident. I had a teacher in Germany named Lucille Heyer. I consider her my most influential teacher because she taught me about the necessity and joy of movement. She was a pupil of Elsa Gindler and she danced with Mary Wigman. Her husband was a psychiatrist and the two of them worked with his patients. Also when I was a little girl I had a dance teacher who instilled in me the joy of movement. She taught until she was in her eighties, and even in her ripe old age she could move very beautifully. Her knowledge of the joy of body movement helped carry her through a difficult life.

The premise of Western medicine is too directed toward the curing of disease, rather than toward prevention. Instead it should teach normalcy: health and how to keep it. It should teach prevention and maintenance. Customarily doctors only get paid and pay attention if you have a disease. But a few well baby clinics have developed which focus on maintaining the health of babies. Kaiser Hospital has one. The children are checked; the mothers are advised; and a symptom is caught before it becomes severe. There should be well grown-up clinics too. Holistic health centers may begin to fill this kind of need. There are some conditions, of course, where you do need a good surgeon, a good orthopedist, or a good internist. But even these specialists could work with the concept of wellness.

## Dance

The differences in treatments for people of different ages are small. Once a person walks, once they dance, after three years of life it is all more or less the same. I watched a lot of children's classes when I was in Sweden. People of different ages move in the same ways, although kids can often move more easily than adults.

I grew up in Nuremburg, Germany, and took my schooling there through the equivalent of two years of college here. Then I went to Munich to do training in breathing, relaxation and movement with Mrs. Heyer whose work was very inspiring. Later in Sweden I worked on many dancers, so I got to know dancers' bodies. They were often tense even though they were moving all the time because their movement was too controlled. A very good dancer moves in a relaxed and easy way. If you have ever seen the Bolshoi Ballet and some of their best dancers, you do not see any effort when they dance. I guess Nijinski was that way. When you dance with ease, contraction and relaxation play into each other. Much dance is mainly contraction, which causes body problems. Alternating contraction and relaxation is the key to prime functioning. You have to release to the same amount that you control in order to create equilibrium. In San Francisco at the Opera House last winter, I saw a dance choreographed by Twyla Tharp. It was gorgeous and different from much modern dance in that even though it was very stylized the movements looked like water. Kathryn Dunam's group was fluid and exuberant also. You go to watch because it passes on this inspiration.

I teach people about breathing mainly through movement. I use the word "breathing" very sparingly in my classes and when I do it is at the end of a session after the participants have relaxed and you see the movement of breathing going through their bodies. Then I say, "Become aware of what happens from the movement in your body." If I told them what to do beforehand it would interfere with their natural release because they're supposed to allow rather than will this movement. I start the classes with slow movements and then we go faster. As we are ending I slow down the pace gradually. Because you need more air as you exercise, you have to become softer, to breathe, to expand your chest and let the diaphragm go down to make room for the lungs to expand.

My exercises would be appropriate warm-ups for athletes and dancers—and for mechanics—for anybody who does anything. If they do these before they work they will be able to perform any activity better.

## Health

The body has an endless longing to improve and to work. If you give the body half a chance, it will get better. One never should say, "I will always have a disability." It need not be so! Many things are apt to get better when you allow yourself to move. I have had people with diagnoses of incurable, congenital difficulties. But with proper movement they lost their aches and pains. If you are willing to give up the idea that a problem is hopeless, your body usually follows suit after a while.

Pleasurable movement, you know, is totally different from forced movement. People say, "Should I do this exercise ten times?" I say, "Do it a few times and feel good; then stop." It is most important to become aware of the pleasure of doing it, not just the duty of doing it. At first, you may do it because you have to, but later as you get the feel of it, it becomes pleasurable. And that is when it serves the body.

What I want to teach in my classes is the way to move with wholeness. A physical therapist usually has excellent knowledge of the body. But I wish physical therapists were allowed to use their knowledge more for prevention, instead of working with people only after their problems have become severe. The more physical therapists could be allowed to work in schools or at colleges to instruct people for healthy daily living instead of having to wait until people come to the hospital and have to pay a lot of money for their services, the better off we would all be because more people would be well. Prevention is also more efficient. You can teach it in a group. You really have to work with sick people individually. I wish insurance companies would insure people and companies for health rather than sickness.

Keeping people in good health is gratifying. It is discouraging to see people only after their health has gone. I've noticed also that people lose weight through doing exercises and moving easily when the whole body is engaged in every movement. It's amazing to see how slender people get and how good they look without any diet. It's not really complicated. If people would simply move their whole bodies, they would feel good.

Enjoyment of the movement is a key part of it. Often people who work too hard forget the pleasure of simple agility. To move smoothly for a long time is enjoyable. Some of the women in my classes in their seventies tell me that they have hiked all over Europe and that it was easy. Then I feel that my teaching is well done, because this is the way it's supposed to be.

# Warm Up: A Flexibility Program

## Preparing

Start the day luxuriously by taking care of yourself first. Find a quiet place in your home with enough room to lie down on a comfortable mat on the floor. The exercise area should be flat and smooth so you can move easily. Be sure you have the privacy you want, so that you don't have to worry about being interrupted.

Begin your routine with a posture check. Simply stand and check your alignment and how your body feels in the morning. Are there any places where you feel stiff?

Then, starting with your feet, check the position of your body. Your feet should be facing forward, and approximately as far apart as your shoulders.

Be sure you're not locking your knees. Bend your knees slightly to take some pressure off your calves and thighs.

Then check your abdomen and your pelvis to be sure that your stomach isn't sticking out and that your pelvis is slightly tucked under.

Beginning at the base of your spine, move your awareness up your spine to see if it feels as though each vertebra is stacked comfortably on top of the other. *In correct, fully erect posture, a line dropped from the ear should go through the outer tip of the shoulder, middle of the hip, back of the knee cap, and front of the ankle.*

When you come to the region of your upper back and chest, be sure that you're not bent forward and hunched in your chest. If you are, inhale and rotate your shoulders back to open up your chest, so that your upper back is not bent and your chest is not caved in. Be sure you're not leaning forward with your neck, and that your chin is tucked under.

When you move you may notice that one side of your body will be loose and more relaxed than the other. See if that is consistent down the full length of your body. My right side is generally slightly tense, and, therefore, less strong and flexible than my left.

As you move, your circulation should pick up and you should feel more awake. Warming up for your exercises is important for good body tone, for preventing strains, and for an enjoyable exercise session. If you start with very vigorous exercise too quickly after you've been asleep or after a day of sedentary work, you'll be working against the condition of all of your muscles, which makes it more likely that you'll strain a muscle.

As you stand, try to imagine that there is a line running from the center of the top of your skull through the center of your body down the length of your spine to the ground. This is the axis of all your movement. Imagine your limbs and muscles move around it as you exercise.

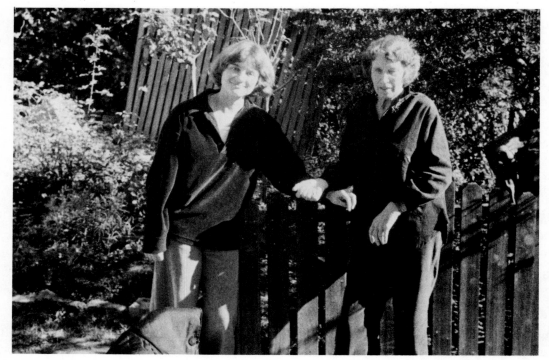

Marion Rosen and Sara Webb

# Marion Rosen's Flexibility Exercises

This is a good point to begin doing Marion Rosen's exercises. Rosen has put together a series of movements to loosen up every joint in your body. You need to move the joints in your body or the synovial fluid will dry up, which causes your joints to become tense and tight. Moving them even a tiny bit each day keep your joints producing this fluid, which keeps the joints flexible.

### Shoulder Jog

Begin with the "shoulder jog." Standing, bend your arms at the elbows, and bring one arm forward while the other goes back. Move at the shoulder as though you were jogging, but only move your arms. Move with your breathing so that you inhale as one arm goes back, and exhale as it comes forward.

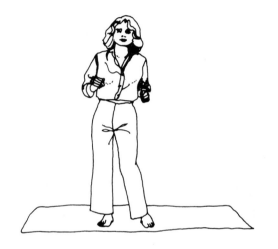

### Stretch Up

Then raise your arms over your head. Inhale; look at the ceiling; stand up on your toes, and reach with both arms, stretching your fingers as high as you can toward the ceiling so that you open up your rib cage and really stretch your back upward. Exhale and relax.

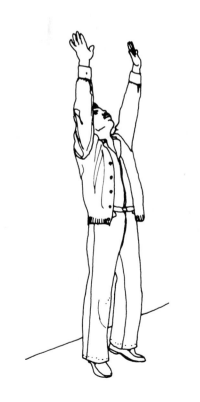

### Hitch Hike

Stand with your weight on your right leg, and your knees slightly bent. Let your left leg relax. Make a circling hitchhiking motion with your right arm so your shoulder rotates. Repeat this on the other side.

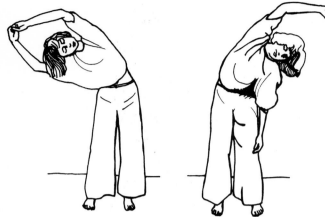

### Side Bender

Inhale. Keep your feet about shoulder width apart. Let your arms relax at your sides. Exhale and bend from your waist toward the left. Be sure that you don't lean forward, but to the side over your hip. Bring your right arm slowly up over your head and let it move to the left in a relaxed arc. Let your head and neck relax toward the left also. This will open up that difficult-to-reach area around your rib cage, from your hips to your shoulders. Inhale as you come to the center again. Relax your arms at your sides. Now repeat this exercise with your other arm, leaning toward the right.

### Wing Rock

This exercise is similar to the "shoulder jog." Bend your arms at the elbows. Stand in a comfortable position. This time bring your elbows out to the side, up toward the ceiling. Now raise one elbow higher as you lower the other. You can feel that this motion moves the muscles around your shoulder blade. Check your knees to be sure that they are still gently bent and your legs are comfortable.

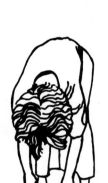

### Hang Loose

Lean forward with your knees bent. Relax your spine and neck and let your arms hang toward the floor. It's important to keep your knees bent so that you don't strain your back. Be sure to let your neck fully relax. You can shake your head a few times to loosen your neck and shoulders. Let your arms hang. This position could be a warm-up for touching your toes. But now you're simply relaxing. Let your arms swing and rotate and feel how this gently opens your upper back around your shoulder blades.

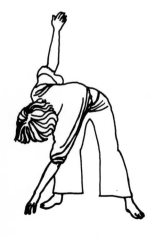

### Bend and Stretch

Spread your feet wider apart than your shoulders, keeping your pelvis tucked under. Inhale. Spread both arms out to the side. Exhale as you lean to your left and touch your left toe with the fingertips of your right hand. Inhale as you stand up again. Next exhale, lean over and touch your right toe with the fingertips of your left hand.

While you're doing this exercise make sure your head and neck are relaxed forward, so that you're not straining by holding your head and looking up. You should be looking down at your toes and breathing as you move. If it's difficult for you to touch your toes, help yourself by bending your knees even more. Gradually the movement will become comfortable so you can do it with your knees just slightly bent.

## Hip Swing

Place your feet farther apart than your shoulders, bend your knees, and squat slightly. Bend your arms at the elbows and rotate your hips in one direction as you move your shoulders in the other while facing forward. It's like dancing the Twist. Inhale as you twist to one side and exhale as you twist to the other. Do this movement a few times. When you're rocking on your feet your knees will rotate from side to side too. I find that this movement helps open up the muscles around my rib cage and the area around the diaphragm, which can be very difficult to relax. This relaxation is critical because the diaphragm is the center of our breathing.

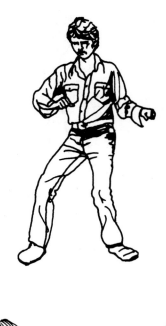

## Pelvic Rock

Place your right foot behind your left foot; straighten out your left leg, and push your pelvis back. Then rock forward so that your weight goes onto your left foot as you move your pelvis forward and lean your torso back. Inhale as you shift your weight forward. Press your pelvis forward as you lean your torso back. Exhale as you shift your weight onto your back foot and bend your torso. Then switch the position of your feet so that your right leg is straight and forward and your weight is on your left foot. Repeat the exercise from this stance.

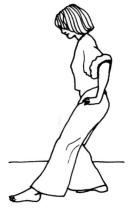 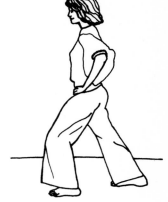

## Knee Swing

Stand with your knees slightly bent and your feet shoulder width apart. Simply swing both knees from side to side as you breathe.

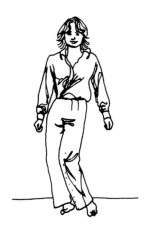

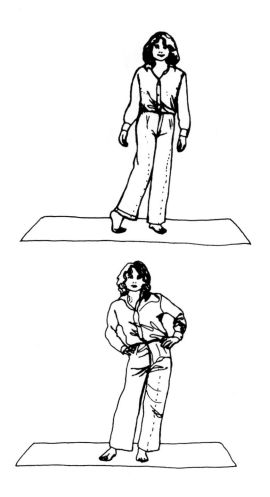

## Heel and Toe

This motion loosens the muscles in your foot and ankle. Stand on your left foot, keeping your right heel on the ground. Point the toes of your right foot toward your left foot. Then pivot on your right heel, so that the toes of your right foot point to the right. Repeat this motion several times with one foot. Switch and stand on your right leg and make the motion with your left foot.

Do this next movement with your weight on one leg also. Place the toe of your left foot on the ground so that the left heel is raised up. Point your left heel toward your right toe. Now pivot on the ball of your left foot so that your left heel is pointing out away from your body and your left knee comes in toward your right knee. Repeat for other side.

## Hip Circles

Rotate your pelvis laterally in full circles in one direction and then another. Breathe in sync with your movement.

## Rest

At this point lie down and rest. Be conscious of your movement as you lie down so that you move from a standing position to a reclining one with as little stress and strain as possible. Try moving toward the floor by bending your knees and leaning forward slightly at the waist. Then let your palms touch the floor as you move into a squatting position. Place your hands on the floor to your right and put your weight on them. Then lie down on your side first. Next roll over onto your back. It's preferable to lie down on your side first, because if you lower your torso to the floor backward from a sitting position, you can strain your back.

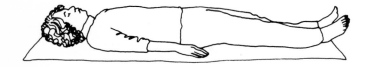

## Knee Flops

After resting a moment, another series of exercises done lying down begins. Begin by bringing your arms up behind your head like a sunbather, with your palms under your head and your elbows out, keeping the small of your back on the floor. Be sure not to arch your back in this position. Inhale and bend your knees. Now exhale as you let your knees fall to the right. Inhale as you bring both your knees up to the center again. Exhale and let your knees and hips roll to the left. Inhale as you come to the center. Repeat this cycle several times.

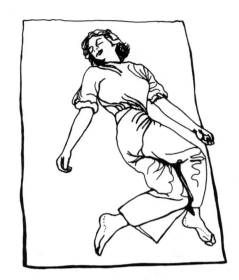

## Side Leg Lift

Roll onto your side; align your spine and your body so that you're not arched at the waist or along your back. Rest your head on your extended arm. Place the palm of your other arm in front of your chest for balance. Inhale and lift both legs off the floor a comfortable few inches at a time. Be sure that when you lift your legs you don't bring them forward, and that you're keeping your body in a straight line. Roll over and do the same exercise on the other side.

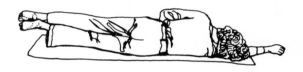

## Straight Leg Circles

Lie flat on your back. Inhale as you lift both legs up and draw large circles in the air with your feet, keeping your legs straight. Do two or three circles to one side, and then to the other.

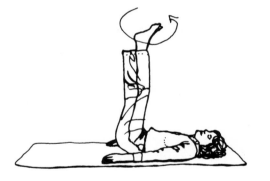

## Sit Ups

Lie flat on your back. Inhale as you raise your torso to a sitting position and reach your arms toward your toes. Let your head and neck relax forward in the process and don't strain. Do it as easily, slowly and comfortably as you can. Exhale as you lower your torso back to the floor.

If you're in very good shape, you can do a shoulder stand, but there are very few backs for

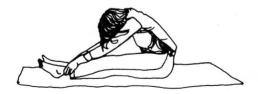

which this exercise is comfortable, or recommended. If you raise your legs and spine off the floor into a shoulder stand, be sure to help support your spine by placing your elbows on the floor and your palms on your back at the waist. Also after a shoulder stand I recommend always arching your back in the opposite direction to balance the stress.

### Final Rest

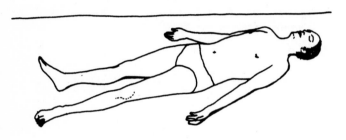

Lie down on your back, relaxing your whole body. Notice how you feel as a result of doing these warm ups and see if your body doesn't feel more alive, more sensitive, and softer.

Marion Rosen's exercises are useful as warm up movements for more vigorous exercise. They are also wonderful if you're in a hurry and don't have time to do a longer exercise routine because they stimulate all the joints in your body and make all the basic movements that you need to loosen up for the day.

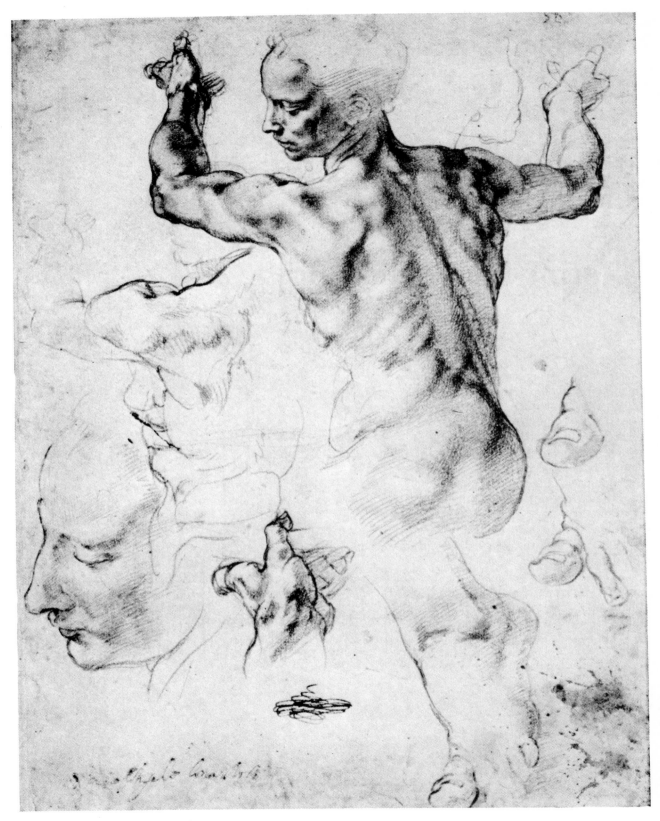

The Libyan Sibyl, Michelangelo

# Testing for Weak Points

Whether you have an injured spine or a healthy one, you probably have one or two spots in your back that are less flexible and slightly weaker than others. You most likely know which parts of your back are stronger than others, and where you feel tension more. In your daily movements, notice which parts of your body, especially in your back that you don't move, and begin to use them. It's important to do some strengthening and loosening of these areas so that they won't become problem centers, and to strengthen muscles in other areas of your body to avoid overburdening your back muscles.

These test postures also make excellent exercises for strengthening the weak area. Practice them over time until they become easy and comfortable.

## The Hips

You need to have strong hip joints and leg muscles to take excess strain from lifting off your back muscles. You can test to see whether you have weak hip flexer muscles by this exercise. Lie on your back on the floor; place your hands behind your neck, and keep your legs straight. Raise both legs about ten inches off the floor, and hold this position for about ten seconds. If this is difficult for you, then do any of the exercises in this book which involve leg lifts.

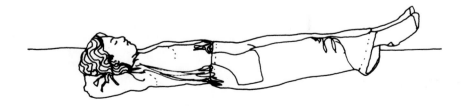

### The Lower Back

You can test for weakness in your lower back muscles by lying on the floor on your stomach and lifting your legs off the floor, keeping your hands clasped behind your head. If you have any difficulty with that movement, then you should do several exercises for strengthening your lower back muscles. All the leg-lifting exercises help develop your lower back. Sit ups are good for strengthening your lower back also, as is the "cow-cat" exercise.

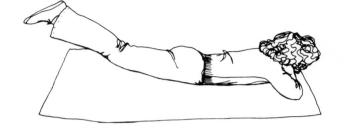

### The Abdomen

Strong abdominal muscles help prevent lower and middle back strain by supporting your body weight in front. If you think your abdominal muscles are weak, try sit ups. If sit ups are difficult for you, then you can do other exercises for your abdominal muscles. Any leg lifts and knee bends are good for this purpose. The "cow-cat" exercise is good for strengthening your abdomen. Use your breathing to strengthen your belly. You can emphasize the contraction and release of your stomach muscles as you exhale and inhale.

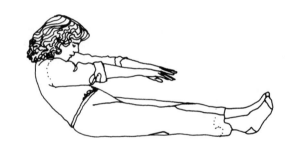

### The Upper Back

If you think your upper back muscles may be weak, test for this by lying on your stomach with a pillow under your abdomen, keeping your thighs, your feet and pelvis on the floor. Raise your torso off the floor with your hands behind your head so that you're using your upper back muscles, not your arms to lift your body. If this is difficult, then you need to do several exercises a day to strengthen and limber your back muscles. All the exercises which involve arching, such as the Fish and the Kneeling Ballet, as well as shoulder strengthening exercises are good for this purpose.

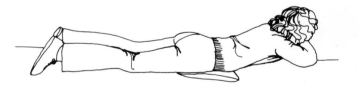

\*   \*   \*

When you have discovered the relative functioning of different areas of your back and related muscles, emphasize exercises of the weak areas in order to balance your strength.

\*   \*   \*

# Prevention Exercises

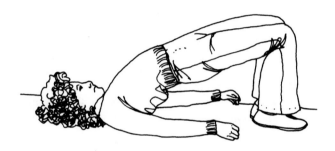

After you have done Marion Rosen's exercises you can do the following exercises for preventing back strain. They are focused on loosening and strengthening the specific areas of your body that connect to critical points on your back. They are simple and can be done almost anywhere. They will teach you to maintain your back in the proper alignment and to make your movements smooth. Variations of these exercises are recommended in almost every back program. They are also good warm up exercises for more strenuous movement or sports. If you add these exercises to your normal movement routine, you'll be taking excellent care of your body.

## Pelvic Tilt

This exercise is designed to strengthen your abdominal muscles and the gluteal muscles in your buttocks. By doing this you are improving the muscular support for your lower back and, therefore, for all your posture. This exercise also helps flatten swayback or lumbar lordosis. Start by lying on the floor. Bend your knees, keeping your feet flat on the floor. Squeeze the muscles of your buttocks very tightly together as though you're trying to hold a coin between them. Still squeezing your buttocks together, pull in your abdomen so that your lower back flattens against the floor. Hold this position for a count of five. Then relax all your muscles and begin the exercise over again. You can also raise your pelvis

off the floor. You can try flattening your back with your legs extended as you're lying on the floor, or when you're standing up, by flattening your back and leaning against a wall. Be careful not to tense your shoulders or contract your neck as you concentrate on releasing your lower back.

Exhale and lower your pelvis to the floor. It's important to lower your back starting at your upper spine moving vertebra by vertebra down to the floor until you reach your tail bone, and then relax. Otherwise you may have a tendency to drop your pelvis before your spine. This would create an arch in your back and would not be training you in a proper movement pattern. You'll know that you're doing it incorrectly if you begin to move like an inchworm across the floor. If this happens, check the order in which you are lowering your pelvis and spine.

## Lower Back Leg Raise

Stand erect. Inhale as you raise one knee and pull it toward your chest with your hands. Exhale as you release your grip and let your knee move away from your chest and lower your leg to the floor again. Repeat with your other leg. This movement helps loosen back muscles and hamstrings.

A limbering variation is to raise your knee and as you exhale, kick your lower leg out in front of you, toes up and heels pressed out. Make several forward leg thrusts as you exhale. Inhale each time you bend your knee to relax your lower leg and foot. Then make these thrust kicks to the side, and to your rear several times. Keep your standing balance by staring at one spot eye level as you kick.

### Back Curl

Starting on your stomach, as you inhale, raise your head and torso off the ground. Bend your knees and raise both legs up behind you. Reach back and grab your ankles with both hands. Give your back a little extra arch by pulling in opposite directions with your legs and arms, while looking up at the ceiling. Exhale and release this position as you lower your legs and torso back to the floor.

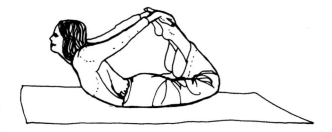

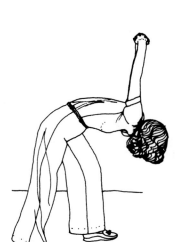

### Upper Back Opener

A really great exercise can be done anywhere, and thus incorporated into your lifestyle. My friend, Satty, confirmed this to me by demonstrating the following exercise in a busy San Francisco bookstore. It's a great release for the upper back and shoulder muscles.

Stand with one foot about twelve inches in front of you, your hands clasped behind you. Keep your rear leg straight. Inhale as you bend the forward leg at the knee and lean your head and torso over your knee; as you do this raise your arms up behind you. Stretch your arms upward so you can feel your shoulder pockets opening and your shoulder blades moving toward each other. Exhale as you lower your arms and stand up straight again. Now bring the back leg forward and repeat this motion bending your other leg.

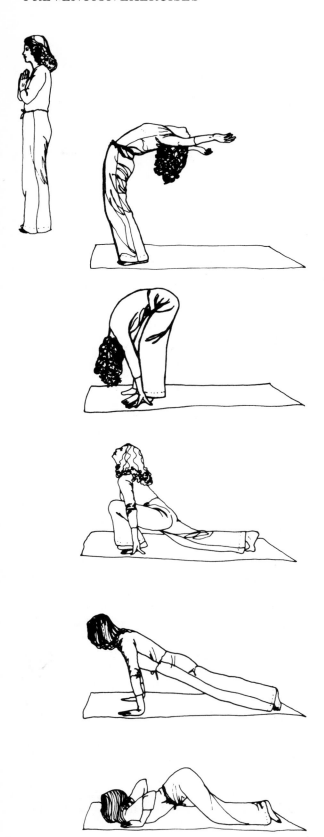

## Salute to the Sun

The single best back exercise I've ever found is a Yoga asana called the "salute to the sun." It's my favorite partly because it's a sequence of movements that feels like a short dance. The sequence exemplifies the most important aspects of good exercise, especially good back exercise. For instance, the sequence in which you do your exercises is important. You should alternate stretching with curling up. By exercising complementary muscle groups, you won't get musclebound. Rather you maintain balanced muscle tone, and the widest possible range of movement and flexibility. In the salute to the sun your breathing is combined perfectly with your movement. The movement sequence is called Soorya Namaskar. Traditionally, the exercise has twelve spinal positions so that you move your spine in every way possible. The sequence is traditionally practiced twelve times in the morning as you repeat the twelve names of the sun. I found that it's not necessary to do the salute to the sun as often as twelve times. Once, when I had sciatica, I did the exercise three times in the morning and three times in the evening, and after two weeks my sciatica was gone. Doing the salute to the sun at least three or four times each morning and evening would keep your spine in wonderful shape. Only do each position as far as it feels comfortable until you loosen up.

Begin the sun exercise in a standing position. Check your spinal alignment and bend your knees slightly. Ideally you should be standing, facing the sun. Fold your hands together; bend your elbows; press your thumbs slightly against the center of your chest.

Inhale as you raise your arms up over your head. Arch your neck and look up at the ceiling; then bend backward so that your whole body makes a round curve.

As you exhale, bend and slowly bring your arms and torso forward and let your whole body relax toward the floor, keeping your neck and head relaxed. When you begin doing this exercise, simply hang in a relaxed position, hands nearly touching the floor. Eventually you want to be able to put both your palms on the ground by your feet and to touch your head to your knees.

In the next position you inhale, extend your arms forward and lean your weight onto them as you extend your right leg straight behind you. Your left knee remains bent and between your hands. Then arch your back and look up at the ceiling.

Now extend your left leg behind you beside your right leg. Inhale; then hold your breath and make your body a straight line from your head down through your spine to your toes, keeping your knees off the floor and your feet together.

Now exhale and lower your torso to the floor, touching your knees down first, then your chin, and then your chest, so that you're curled like a dragon, with your pelvis arched back, and your elbows up in the air. In this position you have eight curves in your body, and the only portions touching the floor are your feet, knees, hands, chest, and forehead.

Now inhale as you flatten your abdomen against the floor; arch your back; and look up at the ceiling.

As you exhale, bring your body up into an arch, keeping your heels, feet and palms flat on the floor, your neck and head relaxed downward.

At this point you have completed the major cycle of the exercise and now will repeat the movements in reverse order to come back to the starting position.

Inhale and lean your weight forward onto your arms and hands, and draw your left foot forward with your knee bent, bringing the foot up between your hands. Arch your back and look up at the ceiling.

Then as you exhale bring your right leg also forward between your hands and lean your torso forward, bringing your head toward your knees. Always keep your knees slightly bent.

As you inhale, arch backward as you did at the beginning of the exercise; raise your arms over your head and bend backward. End by exhaling and relaxing your arms at your sides.

You can begin the exercise again from this point and repeat the whole sequence without pause. You'll find that the next sequence you do will be much easier and more fluid because you'll be loosened up and more relaxed. See if you can get to the point where you move smoothly from one position to the other as though you were dancing, with your breath moving your muscles.

After you've completed the sun exercise, lie down on the floor on your back; relax your arms and legs; close your eyes, and rest a few minutes.

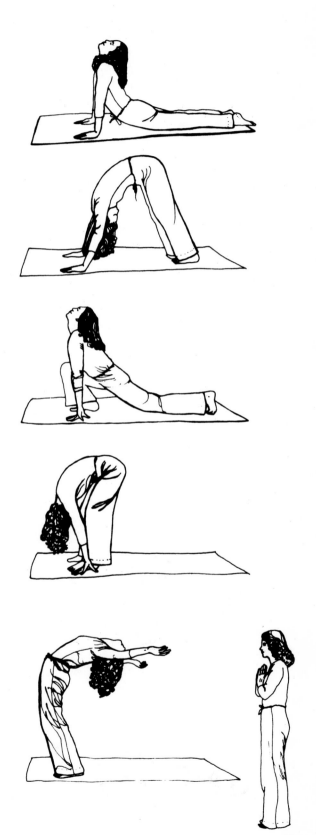

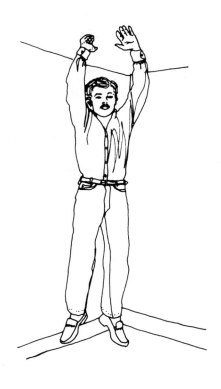

### Jump!

Strengthening your leg muscles and keeping your hip and knee joints flexible are both basic to good back care, because strong legs can prevent extra strain on the back. Jumping is good for limbering and strengthening leg muscles as well as improving your aerobic capacity. It is also fun and a release in the midst of more restricted movements. For the gung-ho jumper, indoor trampolines are available. Also jumping rope is excellent exercise. And jogging on soft surfaces is invigorating.

Or you can make yourself a jumping obstacle course. Place pillows on the floor equal distances apart. Keeping your legs together as you jump, hop over each pillow without stopping.

### Upper Back Release

This exercise is one I invented to reach my upper back and neck, which are difficult to exercise, and are usually quite tense. The hip joints, parts of the buttocks, and the lower back also benefit from these movements.

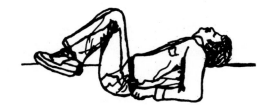

Lie down on your back; bend your knees and draw both legs up to your chest. Prop yourself up on your elbows, so that your knees come toward your forehead. Don't strain; just relax in this position. Now let your head and neck relax backward gradually and sink between your shoulders, so that your shoulders are hunched up. Allow gravity to pull your head backward.

Next let both knees roll sideways. Rotate both legs from side to side, moving your knees toward the floor, and rolling your hips on the floor. Inhale as you bring your knees toward the center; exhale as you move your knees to one side.

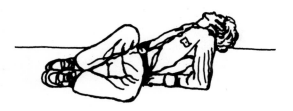

Next add a rotation of your head from side to side. Try moving your head in the same direction that you're rotating the knees, and sometimes in the opposite direction. Also move your shoulders around while your head is resting backward. In this way you can massage the trapezius and upper back muscles that are often difficult to reach. Do these rotations very slowly, but be sure to let the weight of your legs carry your knees all the way to the floor, and give your spine a good, slow, rolling stretch from both ends.

End by bringing your knees back to center, keeping your back relaxed and head sunk between your shoulders. Exhale as you raise your neck and bring your forehead toward your knees.

Then inhale as you relax your whole torso and lower your legs onto the floor. Lie flat and rest.

## The Fish

The fish is the name of a yoga exercise that helps release tension in your upper back, strengthens your neck and your whole spine, and stretches and loosens the muscles of your thighs. Sit on your heels, knees together, and lean your torso back, keeping your knees on the floor. Rest the weight of your torso onto your elbows. Next lower your head toward the floor, relaxing your head and neck backward. Gradually slide your elbows toward your feet so that your torso arches toward the ceiling. Slowly let the top of your head lower to the floor so that eventually you can raise your arms off the floor and let your head and the arch in your back support your torso.

Inhale and raise both arms in a large arc up toward the ceiling, then back over your head. Take a deep breath, opening up your chest and back as you arch. Exhale as you bring your arms back down to your sides. Repeat this arm lifting and breathing sequence several times.

Now slide your knees and feet out from under you. Relax for a moment flat on your back. Then draw your knees up toward your chest. Place your hands on your knees, and lie in that position a little while to give your spine a chance to curl up in the opposite direction to avoid cramping. This curl is a good position to adopt for resting any time between exercises. It takes the pressure off your middle back and helps you learn to flatten your spine against the floor without arching your back.

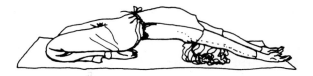

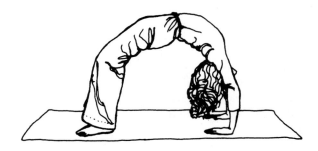

## The Arch

This is one of my favorites, but if you've had any kind of back injury, you probably shouldn't attempt it. If you do have a healthy spine, doing this exercise is a good way to keep yourself limber and to balance out the forward movements that you make more often during the day. Lie flat on your back. Bend your knees and draw your feet as close to your buttocks as possible. Then stretch your arms behind your head and place your palms on the floor with your elbows up toward the ceiling. Pressing your feet down on the floor, inhale and raise your pelvis off the floor. Gradually arch your whole back, pushing up with your hands and feet. Breathe in this position a few seconds. Then lower your body to the floor again by placing your head, neck, spine, and then your pelvis on the ground as you exhale. Then bring your knees toward your chest and rest a few moments on your back in this position.

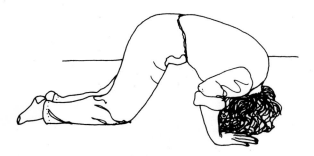

## Neck and Spine Stretch

This exercise is for releasing tight neck muscles. It is a variation of a Yoga spinal stretch. Kneel on a mat or rug. Sit on your heels and exhale as you lean your torso forward, both arms stretched out in front of you. Lower your arms, head and torso to the ground. Rest a few moments in this position, breathing easily so that your pelvis can settle down on your heels to increase the lumbar extensor stretch.

Now inhale and raise up on your hands and knees, keeping your head and neck relaxed down. Then exhale and push your torso forward over your hands by tucking your pelvis under and straightening your thighs, the top of your head on the floor. Allow your body weight to shift onto your arms and head as you lean farther forward, stretching the neck. Very gradually reverse the position as you inhale until you return to the crouch in which you began. Rest a few moments and repeat. This cycle helps relieve headache pain.

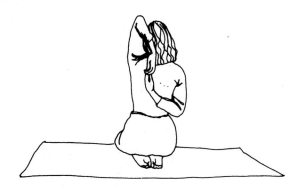

## Headaches and Exercise

Because your spine functions as a whole, constriction of the neck muscles is not the only form of tension which causes headache pain. Tension from tight shoulders, tense upper back muscles, a tilted pelvis, or constricted lower back muscles can work its way up the spine and manifest itself as a splitting headache. When you do any of these back exercises be especially aware of relaxing your neck muscles. Any of the exercises will help relieve the headache, but some of them will focus more on your individual problem areas. Try out the exercises and see which ones reach the muscles in your body whose constriction is usually responsible for your tension headaches. Do your selected neck and back exercises as soon as you feel the beginnings of headache tension. This will prevent the constriction from progressing into full-blown pain. And remember to keep your head aligned with your spine to avoid neck strain while standing or sitting.

## Holding Hands

This exercise opens up the chest and helps release the upper back and shoulder tension that most of us have. Inhaling, bring up your left arm, and then move your left hand behind your back and point your left elbow toward the ceiling. Place your palm over your spine between your shoulder blades. Next, bend your right arm at the elbow, tucking your hand under you, and bring your right arm up behind you, sliding your right hand up your spine to meet your left hand. Then hold hands with yourself behind your back. Breathe and relax in this position for a few seconds. Then release the position slowly, and reverse the position of your arms to repeat the same motion on the other side.

## The Squat

The next position is good for your whole body. In rural America it's often referred to as "The Arkansas squat." In many countries where it is not customary to use chairs, this is the position people sit in all the time. It keeps your hip and knee muscles particularly flexible. Sitting on chairs tends to allow the hip muscles to atrophy. This exercise also helps relax your upper back and your rib cage.

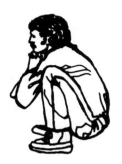

Place your feet flat on the floor, and bend your knees so that your derriere is almost touching the floor. Lean your torso forward; position your shoulders between your knees; and clasp your hands. Rest with your chin on your hands in this position. Or you can take your thumbs, place them on either side of the bridge of your nose near your eye sockets, and rest your forehead forward on your thumbs. If it's comfortable for you, this position can be interesting for meditation.

## Hard Boiled Egg Rock

I like to end my morning exercise with some good stimulation for my spine. This is the movement I use. From a sitting position roll back onto your buttocks. Keep your knees bent; bring your feet off the floor, hugging your knees with both arms; pull your head and neck forward; put your forehead on your knees so you're sitting on your buttocks, resting comfortably.

Then, bring your arms slightly down to your sides so that you're holding your knees with your palms, and tuck your elbows snugly against your legs on either side. Next rock your body backward and forward on your spine as many times as you can comfortably. This exercise is best done on a rug. Inhale as you roll back and exhale as you roll forward. Once as I was doing this exercise, my friend, Charlie Latimer, said I looked like a hard boiled egg rolling in a pot of water. Ever since, this is what it's been like for me. You can use the momentum of the last rock forward to roll onto your feet and into a squat. Then lean your torso forward and stand up. This rolling movement is very stimulating to the nerves in your spine, and is a good way to complete the series of exercises actively.

## Sitting Up Well

Lie down on your back and relax. Then move to a sitting position by rolling over onto your side, bending your knees slightly while bringing them up toward your chest. Roll your weight forward onto your arms and hands, and push yourself up from your side into a sitting position.

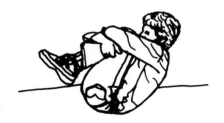

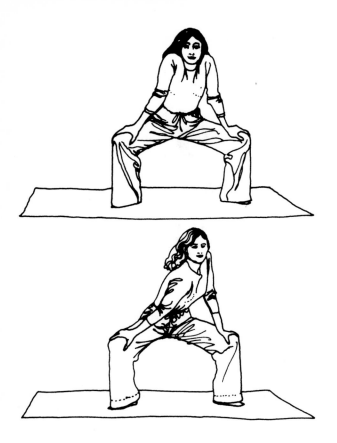

## Cracking Your Back

You might want to try "cracking" your spine. I find one easy way to do that is to incorporate it into the exercise called Upper Back Release. When you move your knees from side to side on the floor, twist your spine more and try to use the weight of your legs to "crack" your spine as you roll.

You can also try cracking your back in a standing squat. Spread your legs widely apart; bend your knees; hunch over with your palms on your knees, so that your shoulders are up toward your ears, and your body weight rests on your hands and arms. Keep your spine and torso facing forward, but as you exhale twist your right shoulder toward your left side so that you can feel a slight pull in your lower spine. Try the same motion with your left shoulder, moving it toward your right side, feeling your vertebrae curl.

It took me several weeks of doing this motion once or twice every day before my spine finally "cracked." Once it did, I had the feel for it; now I can do it easily at any time. Persist!

## Resting

When you feel that your back is strained, even slightly, or that you need to rest for a little while to regain some energy, there are several pleasant rest positions you can use.

One is to lie on your side; draw your knees toward your chest, keeping your head and your spine in a straight line, and fold your arms across your chest and relax.

This next position for resting the spine is more comfortable for some people than for others. Kneel, sitting on your heels and arch your back slightly. Lower the front of your head to the floor. Let both arms hang loosely at your sides, palms up, and see if you can really release your shoulders so that they're hanging toward the floor. Take several deep breaths, so that your whole spine and back open up as you sit in this position.

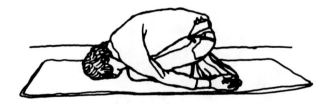

You can use these rest positions in between exercises, to break from any strenuous activity, or at any moment when you feel the need to relax. It's an important part of preventive exercise to assume these relaxing positions from time to time and to treat yourself kindly so that you never overstress.

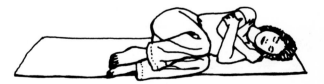

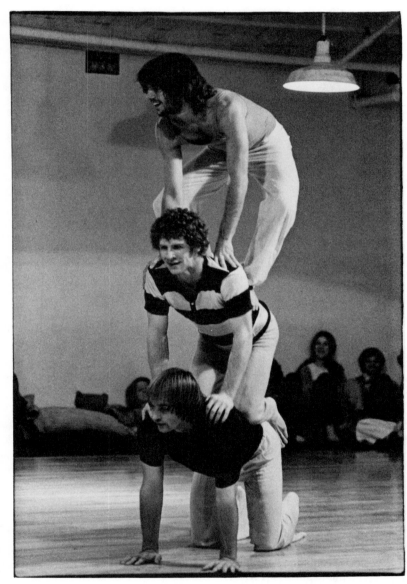

Diane Coleman

# Back to Back:
# Exercises for Couples & Groups

### Back Breathing

This exercise enables two people to tune in to their own backs and their partners' as well. Sit back to back on the floor with your legs crossed. Relax your hands in your lap and close your eyes. Without talking try to arrange your

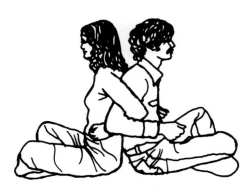

body positions so you can comfortably lean on each other with mutual support and no strain.

Once you've found this position together, tune in to your own breathing and try to relax the rest of your body so that the breath moves deep in your belly. Note the muscles of your back which move in response to your breathing. Notice your partner's back and how it feels leaning against you. See if you can feel the movement of your partner's muscles in his or her back as a result of breathing. Once you have tuned in to your partner's breathing, notice whether you

change your own breathing while searching for your partner's. Did you change your breath pattern to match your partner's without thinking? If such changes happen, see whether you can let your breath relax in your belly again and maintain your own rhythm while being aware of your partner's. The ability to do this is often related to your patterns in daily relationships and the capability to be sensitive to another person's habits while maintaining your own.

A good way to end this exercise is to imagine that you are exhaling through your lower back, as though you could breathe into each other's backs. Let yourself do this awhile and see what sensations arise. Now lock arms at the elbows. Place your feet flat on the floor with your knees bent. See if you can help each other stand up back to back. From the standing position, you can begin the Back Lift.

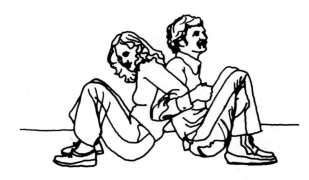

### Back Lift

This exercise is done with one partner in a standing position and the other leaning over backward. Stand back to back and lock arms at the elbows. Bend your knees slightly and squat a little so that your buttocks are just below your partner's. Then slowly lean forward, with your knees bent, until your back gradually becomes parallel with the floor. At the same time your partner should be arching his or her back backward and leaning over onto your back. Hopefully your partner can relax arched on your back, and release his or her spine. This position should be comfortable for both of you with absolutely no strain on the person carrying the weight if your knees are bent and your back is in the correct position. If lifting causes any strain, stop and shift your position. If you are on top, relax and enjoy being lifted by someone else and having the stress taken off your legs and back.

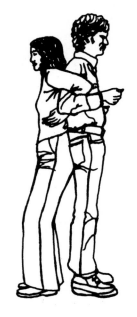

After a minute or so, bend your knees a little more and straighten up to let the person you've been supporting back down so the feet are touching the ground again and your partner can stand up. Alternate positions with your partner and repeat the exercise so you have a turn being lifted.

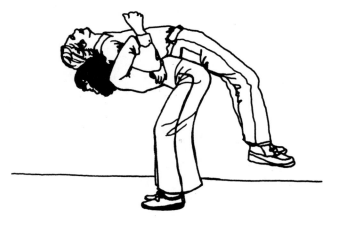

### The Rocking Horse

This exercise is done with two people sitting on the ground facing each other, the soles of their feet touching, legs straight out in front, toes pointing toward the ceiling. Straighten your back and join hands with your partner. Begin a rocking horse motion as one person leans the torso back and the other person leans forward. Exhale as you curl over. Inhale as you lean back. Do this motion slowly, paying attention to your breathing as you rock. Don't push yourselves to the point where you hurt your legs or back. Placing the soles of your feet on the floor and your toes touching your partner's, gradually increase the angle of your rocking so that as you lean forward you almost come to a standing position. As you lean backward, support your standing partner; hold firmly and let your partner return to the floor gradually.

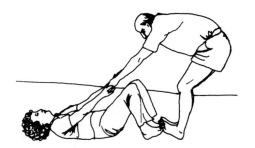

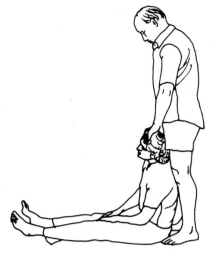

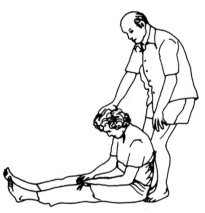

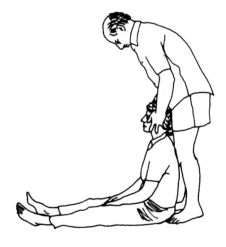

### Help From Friends

In this exercise, one person stands while the other sits down, legs straight out, with his or her back to the partner's feet. The sitting person leans back against the legs of the stander. If you are standing, bend your knees slightly; let your head relax forward; place your palms on either side of your friend's head. Gently move your friend's head from left to right. Ideally, the person sitting on the floor will relax enough so when you are moving their head, they don't tense against the side to side movement. Then help your partner relax her head forward.

If you are standing, next place your palms on your partner's shoulder blades. If you are sitting on the floor, let your back relax and let your neck and head fall forward. Let your whole torso lean toward your legs as you exhale. If you are standing, flex your knees gently to rock the person sitting in front of you. Don't push your friend any farther forward than is comfortable. After a few minutes of rocking, slowly straighten your knees and let your friend sit up. Then place your palms around the back of the skull and let your fingers curl around either side of the jaw. Try raising your friend's head up slightly so that you stretch the neck. If you are sitting down, relax and allow your head to be lifted.

The stretching movement should be smooth and slight so that you do not strain the person's neck. If you are standing, place your palms behind your friend's head and let them lean back to rest the whole head in your hands. Now holding your friend's head in your hands, walk backward and ease him or her down so that your friend can eventually come to a supine position on the floor.

If you are lying down, relax for a while, noting the way your body feels from the exercise. Then trade places with your friend and repeat the exercise.

### Circling

You can do another exercise in the rocking horse position that stretches the muscles of your back. Spread your legs apart comfortably on the floor. Hold hands with your partner and keep the soles of your feet together. Begin the exercise as you did the rocking horse. One person leans forward while the other leans back, supporting each other with your hands and feet. Gradually change your forward motion to a sideways motion so that you both begin to draw large circles on the floor with the movement of your torso. Inhale, lean back and to the right; lean your torso farther to the right as you lean forward; then come to the center. Now make a larger circle moving your head and torso to the left.

Increase the speed of your circling as much as is comfortable. Keep your breathing synchronized so that you inhale as you arch backward and exhale as you drop forward. Going faster and faster can be fun if the position is physically comfortable.

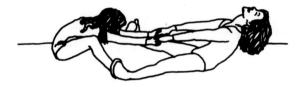

## Spine Cradle

This exercise can be done most effectively with a group of ten or more. One person sits on the floor with his or her back against a wall, the spine straight and comfortable, legs spread out in front of them. A second person sits between the first person's legs, and leans back onto his or her chest. The next person repeats this position, and the next, so that eventually there's a long line of people, each resting their back on the torso of the person behind them. Once the line is formed and comfortable, everyone closes their eyes and relaxes. After awhile you will notice that you're all breathing in unison. Often people experience a deep sense of relaxation from this long line of back support. The exercise can be a soothing way to end a class.

## The Backettes

Marion Rosen, and Sara Webb who often works with her, usually turn their class exercises into group activities. This helps increase the group energy, makes some of the less variable exercises more interesting, and helps integrate the group's rhythm. Almost any exercise that is done standing and moving the legs can be done in groups. People can stand in line with their arms around each other's shoulders and move their legs in time with each other, somewhat like the Rockettes. If the exercise calls for moving across the floor, or jumping, you can form a line by holding hands or move in a circle holding another person's shoulders. You can also do many movements holding hands in a circle as you coordinate your movements with those of the other people around you. It's good to do these kinds of group exercises to music and let its rhythm suggest the rhythm of your exercises.

Back breathing can be done in large groups. Have each back to back couple sit knee to knee with another couple with all the touching couples in a circle. Or the couples can sit side by side in long rows, touching palms with the persons next to them.

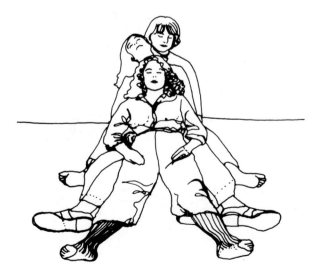

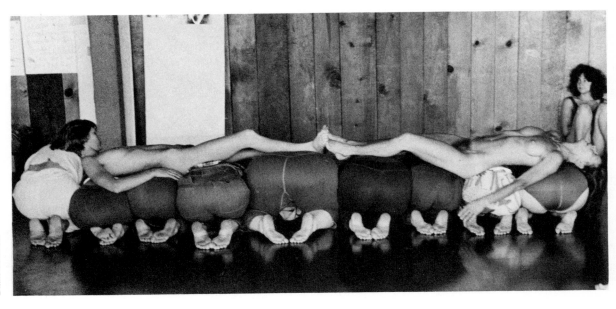

Diane Coleman

83

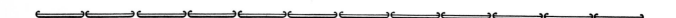

Alice looked pityingly at him. "Tying up the face is very good for the tooth-ache," she said.

"And it's very good for the conceit," added the Wasp.

Alice didn't catch the word exactly. "Is that a kind of toothache?" she asked.

The Wasp considered a little. "Well, no," he said: "it's when you hold up your head—so—without bending your neck."

"Oh, you mean stiff-neck," said Alice.

The Wasp said, "That's a new-fangled name. They called it conceit in my time."

"Conceit isn't a disease at all," Alice remarked.

"It is though," said the Wasp: "Wait till you have it, and then you'll know. And when you catches it, just try tying a yellow handkerchief round your face. It'll cure you in no time!"

—Lewis Carroll, THROUGH THE LOOKING GLASS

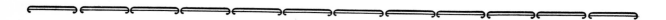

# Emotions & the Back

Because of the interaction of mind and body, we need to be aware of the role of our emotions in our backs' health. Many back problems are the result of chronic daily tensions. Under prolonged stress, the body gives way eventually and the tension earns the new label: "back problem." In considering the correspondence of psychological factors to back tension, we might ask ourselves, "Why would we unnecessarily hold any part of the body tight? Why wouldn't we choose to relax and move freely?" It isn't only the fact that our bodies grow tired as we grow older, because many young people develop back problems, while many older people do not.

Folklore, psychology and medicine all attribute certain emotional content to back problems. Many of our figures of speech reveal our assumptions about the meaning and moods of the back. For instance: "Don't turn your back on me." "You have no spine." "She shoulders too much responsibility." "I need a shoulder to cry on." "It's on your shoulders." "He's flat on his back." "He'll back out on you." "Back off!" "Get back!"

In body therapy analysis the function of a tense body part gives a clue to the cause of the problem. Sexual fears and early childhood anxieties are often causes of lower back problems, as well as being heavy emotional burdens. Unexpressed heartfelt emotions are often held in tense chests and middle back muscles. Tight shoulders are thought to be signs of too much responsibility, unexpressed anger, and/or stifled ambitions. Sadness and fear as well as the tension of unsaid words are sometimes thought to be held in tense throat muscles. A stiff neck is often thought to be a sign of opinionatedness.

Popular generalizations often prove valid. But because each body part has many functions and each person's functioning is individual, relying on the generalizations is dangerous. In so doing a person's unique patterns may be overlooked. So in a psychological analysis it seems more useful to regard a bodily reaction as just one among many corresponding clues which lead to a diagnosis. Whatever its meaning, however, body tension must be cleared up before the psychological problem can be completely healed.

The inseparable connection of physical and emotional tension is a major reason for maintaining full body mobility. It's not only the muscles and joints which benefit from movement; the whole body and psyche are nourished by exercise. When you are properly aligned and flexible, there is more room in your body for the organs, more room for breathing. Breathing affects the circulation of blood to all the organs and tissues in the body. When you learn to move well and easily you not only move beautifully and more functionally, your emotional and psychological tensions are freed from their hiding places in your body and may be integrated and dealt with in the process of living.

Some doctors now refer to a type of individual as having a "backache personality." Ambition is a major giveaway of this profile, especially worldly ambition. To the back-ache personality, work is often an absolute priority, leading to the sacrifice of physical health in order to meet project demands. These people often think of themselves as invincible and have a 'mind over matter' attitude. They also may kid themselves that they are in as good shape now as they were in their youth, when no stress was too much for their available stamina.

Besides seeing themselves as Wonder Women or Bionic Men, backache personalities may also be reluctant to appear socially distraught. Maintaining a cool veneer may seem more necessary than giving in to emotional and physical impulses. Bernard Finneson, M.D., in his book THE NEW APPROACH TO LOW BACK PAIN, has this to say about such sufferers:

> The psychiatrist called upon to assess a patient with low back pain would look into whether the person was under stress...especially...whether the person saw himself as carrying burdens beyond his capacity to bear under circumstances where the struggle involved failed to provide the gratifications which were his due or which he felt were.... These particular low back pain patients are troubled by inner emotional (psychic) struggles over dependency and independence.... They are people who feel pressured beyond their natural point of endurance.... Job-related or marriage stresses often set off backaches in... 'people who are divided—conscientious and yet rebellious at the same time, can't say no to the boss but really can't say yes either.... They have a reluctance to bear burdens cheerfully or with enthusiasm.... They say yes, but they protest with their backs.'[14]

Considering all the problems which may result from holding tension in the back, it would seem wise for us to learn to recognize our emotional symptoms early and relieve their causes before they lead to major illness. If we often have conflicting responses to situations but usually express the most conservative one, perhaps we should find an appropriate place, like a psychologist's pillow or a tennis backboard, to vent the responses that we feel are too negative for our regular society. In this way we can help prevent suppressed anger or frustration from overburdening our lower backs. Heavy exertion sports or strenuous exercise is a valuable outlet for emotions too strong or violent for social exchange. We also need to acknowledge sexual conflicts and deep emotional fears openly to circumvent their becoming pent-up in our muscles.

If we are ambitious, perhaps we can channel that so that, rather than expressing it as a drive to succeed in spite of our bodies' needs, we use it to focus on staying healthy and preventing back problems. Whatever the emotional elements of our body lives, we need to be sure not only to abandon our crutches and fantasies, but also to replace them with productive, healing support images. This way our bodies can become channels enabling us to process almost any stress or surprise.

\* \* \*

**'Know yourself.' It is a difficult task, seductive and painful.**
—Isabelle Eberhardt, THE DIARIES

\* \* \*

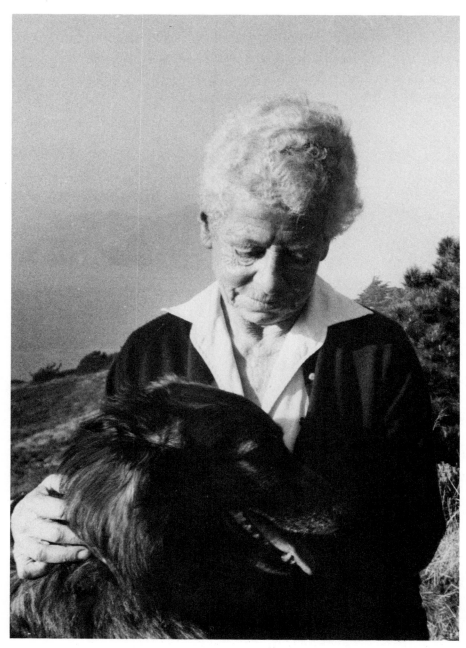

Magdalene Proskauer

# A Therapist: Magdalene Proskauer

Magdalene Proskauer, a graduate of the University of Munich, Germany, received a degree in physiotherapy from the University of Munich Medical School and headed the physiotherapy department of an orthopedic hospital in Munich. She worked in Yugoslavia at the Zagreb City Hospital, in New York at the Presbyterian Medical center for the treatment of polio, cerebral paralysis and posture corrections, and also in Los Angeles. Magda has now settled in San Francisco, where she conducts classes in breath awareness and has a private practice. Magda has developed a precise and powerful therapy combining breathing awareness, movement release and dream analysis. I studied these techniques with her for several years and found her work to be more effective at a deep level than almost any other form of body work I experienced because of its subtlety, gentleness, and focus on long term rather than short term psychological integration. In this chapter, Magda talks about the connections between emotional and physical factors in the treatment of back problems.

## Integrating Mind and Body

I work from the point of view that body and psyche are two aspects of the same reality, two manifestations of the whole personality which are in constant interaction. Our physical behaviour seems to correspond to a psychic pattern of synchronicity. Synchronicity is a meaningful coincidence. If you study the dreams of people with back trouble you can find clues to the psychological correspondence with the back problem. At times after the back gets better, we find out what the problem's psychological meaning was. So when there is back trouble I treat the symptom first. When the physical problem is gone, very often the psychological problem surfaces.

We can approach our problems both ways, physically and psychologically. The psychotherapist tries to bring the problem into consciousness through psychotherapy; the physical therapist works by approaching the body. We have to learn to take care of our weaknesses. Whenever we regress a little or fall back into an old pattern, the physical problem may come back again. And even if you know the psychological problem, you have to treat the back.

In the spine the lower back is the problem for most people, usually the fifth lumbar vertebra and the first sacral vertebra, between the L5 and S1. Those areas often become disintegrated or herniated. I first go through the conventional path of having a doctor make an x-ray to diagnose what is harmed to discover if there is arthritis, if there is a disintegrated vertebra, or whatever. When we know what is wrong we treat it.

When people are really in pain, the first phase of recovery is bed rest. The reason why doctors put people into the hospital in traction is often so they simply can't get out of bed. At home people get impatient and after a while get up. But in the hospital they stay put.

The psyche often needs a rest too. Psychologically there are reasons why you are flat on your back. Some people always fall flat on their backs because they don't have 'enough spine.' Some people are too driven to submit to rest. What we call the negative animus can lead one to go against one's self as a woman, or be too opinionated, or not able to assert oneself enough. We speak of people that 'don't have a spine' when they are without structure and persistence.

Rest is the very first phase of recovery. Then comes mild exercise. Many people exercise too much too soon. When a doctor gives them a sheet of exercises, they go home, and if they are conscientious they do them all right away. Then they're on their backs again because the muscles have become so weak from resting that they can only be built up again slowly. Very gently you should start to strengthen the abdominal muscles first. When you strengthen the abdominal muscles the back muscles have a chance to go into balance. Then you build what we call a muscle corset, so that all muscles are in balance.

The moment you get back problems the back muscles go into spasm, the abdominal muscles get flabby and the back often gets bent even more. So I work very gently. My exercises aim at loosening each part of the body and raising the muscle tone.

When people are well again they really have to take responsibility for themselves and to acknowledge what they can and can't do; not lifting or knowing how much they can lift, for instance. They have to exercise every single day, and the best exercise is swimming. I myself have a deteriorated disc so I swim every day in a pool warm enough so that the muscles don't go into spasm when suddenly the weather temperature goes down. There is a tremendous amount of preventive care possible.

I haven't seen many operations which were successful unless a disc was herniated and had to be operated on to relieve the pressure on the nerves. Most other problems you should be able to take care of by exercise, rest and becoming aware of the area so that you feel the problem before it gets bad. It's also important to eat well and not to gain weight so that there's no extra weight to carry around. The concept of doing something preventive to maintain well being, that is, the preventive approach to medicine, and also to other parts of life, before you have the problem, is the concept that most people don't have at all. The person who has back trouble has to lie down before he or she gets a back ache. After a long car or plane trip, even without having pain, they should lie down with the legs propped up, so that the back can rest, before it starts to hurt. It is a tremendous education. Not everybody learns to live preventively, but when they learn they're o.k.

I have one case right now of a woman who was operated on after a car accident. She was in agony and it took a long time for her to really learn to live a new way. Now for over a year she has been traveling and everything is fine. She is very careful. She swims every day. She does her exercises. She's an artist so she sometimes stands on ladders to work but she knows when she has to lie down. She learned to adjust. But some people don't want to change their life. They want the doctor to give them a pill. There is no pill. We're only human beings. We make mistakes. But every time the backache returns, it can be a learning experience.

That's why I say there is a meaning to symptoms. One of the meanings is to accept your limitations. You learn what you can do with your body and what you cannot. For instance, jogging is not good for everybody. Some people jog for the back, but too much jogging isn't good. Some jogging might be fine, on the beach, on soft surfaces. But to jog on hard streets is bad for your back. Many people have compressed spines from jogging. They also get very stiff, probably because they overdo it or they don't warm up enough.

Certain areas of the back may manifest specific problems. A stiff neck, for example, may indicate stubbornness. The prophets in the Old Testament mediate the word of God, saying, 'I will not dwell among you stiff-necked people any longer.' In modern language this means the self-willed people did not follow the voice of God, their inner voice. Ego-centered and opinionated attitudes often go together with a stiff neck, but not always. You can have a whiplash in a car accident cause a stiff neck. The stiff neck also has to do very often with the intellectual attitude. When people start to read a lot early in life in a bad posture the neck sometimes becomes contracted, and later on in life they get stiff necks and stiff shoulder muscles.

But I'm always careful not to say, 'This symptom goes with this psychological problem,' because problems are pretty individual. Stomach ulcers are often connected with being overambitious. But it's dangerous to make absolute statements. All you can do is observe, when you work on the body, what the psychological problem might be. Most people who get these problems are not in their bodies enough. You correct the problems some with more body awareness.

Also your discs can degenerate if you are born with weak, thin discs. You may not feel it until you are in your forties or fifties. I was in a car accident, and that was when I felt the weak point in my back for the first time. When I observed my x-rays, I saw that the lumbar discs were quite weak, which I had never known because I always exercised so much. I also found out, when I was over sixty, that I had some spurs in my spine. I never felt that when I was younger because I did a lot of exercises and never had trouble.

I think I probably overdid horseback riding. I was jumping horses and played a tremendous amount of tennis. I was very athletic and could carry heavy loads. Since I never had back trouble, I probably used up my discs, not knowing that they were weak.

I swim every day, at the moment forty-five minutes. I have a Jacuzzi at home. Every morning I do my exercises for ten or fifteen minutes and I take a Jacuzzi. On my lunch hour I go swimming. It's an outdoor heated pool and I take another Jacuzzi there, dry myself in the sauna five minutes, exercise again a few minutes and then I'm fine again. One has to be careful when swimming. It is better not to do the breast stroke because you can strain your lower back by lifting your head. When you have back trouble you should swim side strokes, back strokes and the crawl. Swimming exercise, like all exercise, should be mild, not pushing. You should swim gently in the water long enough to loosen all the muscles. The secret to the benefit of swimming is that you are nearly weightless and, therefore, the spine moves without having so much gravity pull and weight on it. First you have to be without pain or at least with very little, and then swimming does the most for your back. I started with five or ten minutes a day, then twenty minutes, then half an hour, then forty-five minutes. You have to pace yourself daily according to your condition.

## Visualization

People have to understand what is happening in their bodies to reap the most benefit from exercise. That is the reason I use visualization. Now Dr. Simonton in Texas is doing visualization work with cancer patients. He tells them to visualize how the cancer can be swept away, and it helps. He also gives them medication and chemotherapy. His comparative studies show that patients who use visualization along with his other treatments get better results than the patients who do not use visualization. I show my clients their x-rays. I make drawings of how the spine looks. I show them how the space between the vertebrae opens in movement. If you can visualize it, you can feel it better. When you feel it, it works better than if you just do it mechanically. If you do it mechanically, you make mistakes. You don't really release.

You have to be aware and feel what you do in order for the exercise to work well. That's why the mechanical exercises, or those done too fast, contract muscles instead of release tension. It's also easy to strain again unless you are very subtle in your movements. The visualization is encouraged by the particular kind of breathing that I teach. For instance, I ask you to breathe as if the breath were spreading in the pelvis. One movement is to contract and release the buttocks. I describe the hip joints to you as you move. I tell you the hip joint is made of a ball and socket. The socket part is created by the pelvis. The ball is the top of the thigh bone. When we are tense we pull our legs too far into the hip joint. When we can release our tension the leg can come slightly out of the joint, and we created a little space between the socket and the ball. I talk anatomy to help you visualize it exactly. By visualizing this, it can actually happen that the hip joint loosens up.

Then I say, 'Feel the hip while you exhale.' Some people can feel the hip joints. Then I make a short cut and I say, 'Exhale into the hip joints.' This is impossible, but it's a helpful image. It really *feels* as if you can send your breath into the hip joints. I talk to the body directly. That makes you visualize the situation, and when you visualize it, you can reach it better. You can feel it better.

I also give instructions to pause after the exhalation until the direct inhalation happens by itself. This helps to find our genuine rhythm. We breathe unconsciously or automatically from the moment we are born. We can also breathe consciously; we can stop breathing a while and change our breath at will. The breath is like a bridge between the unconscious and conscious nervous systems. You can't contract your stomach or other organs consciously. You usually only feel them when you are in pain. Because the breath is connected with the conscious and the autonomous (unconscious) nervous systems, it forms a bridge between them. When you focus on the breath you make a normally unconscious function conscious.

You can use your breathing to make other unconscious functions more conscious. By focusing on the breath you may get in touch with certain unconscious emotions, for instance. That's why people sometimes cry when they start to relax from deep breathing. Dreams are an unconscious product, but if you remember the dream when you wake up, you bring this unconscious message into consciousness, and you can learn to understand what it wants to tell you.

Some people even have visions during my exercise classes; some people don't. Jung encouraged people in what he called 'active imagination,' which is to concentrate in order to find one's images, but there are people who can't. Others can learn active imagination. Some people dream but can't remember their dreams. They are cut off from the unconscious. It's a very natural state to be in touch with your unconscious, but in our society there are many people that don't have visions or dreams. Some people can renew their contact with the unconscious by doing special breathing exercises.

## Staying With the Body

It's an education to deal with your back pains. You must wear comfortable shoes. No high heels. Many people have back problems due to wearing the wrong shoes. And many people get back problems from exercising—that is, exercising incorrectly. Very young, very flexible people can, of course, do anything. But if there is a slight hint of a back problem, yoga back bends are not good. They increase the lumbar curve, extend the abdominal muscles and contract the back muscles. We want the opposite for a healthy back.

The lumbar area seems to be a weak point in our structure. We no longer walk on all fours but our bodies have not adjusted perfectly to standing upright. A baby is born with a completely straight spine. When the baby sits up, slowly the neck curve develops to hold the head up. Then they start crawling. And when they start to stand up, the lower back curve develops fully.

The place of the balance for our bodies is in the lower back. I think we're not quite structurally meant to walk upright because we're not quite developed at the curve in the lower spine. With a curve in the spine there is a chance for it to compress the vertebrae there. If the vertebrae get compressed, the disc, which is like a shock absorber, gets pressed together and pinches the nerves, which causes pain. So we have to be careful with our spines and with how we move and live.

In healing a back problem one needs all the physiological and psychological information available. Many people today get too psychological, and that's again an escape from the body. They say, 'Oh, I know *why* I have my backache.' Even if it is true, that isn't enough to solve the back problem. You cannot run away from the body. You have to stay with the body in order to cure it.

# Visualization

The value of visualization, long a healing method used in ancient systems of thought such as Yoga, Shamanism and witchcraft, is beginning to be recognized by some branches of modern medicine. One method frequently used in yoga is to see yourself doing a movement in your mind's eye before actually making it with your body. Such previsualization seems to be a kind of practice which gives the effect of doing a movement twice. Dr. Carl Simonton and his wife Stephanie in Texas are gaining renown for their successful treatment of cancers by encouraging their patients to use visual imagery of their bodies becoming healthy, along with other treatment, to stimulate their healing.

Visualization is a good form of healing for people who are too sick or injured to perform exercises. It also can be a powerful addition to your physical routine, one which can help improve your image of your health. Visualization can be done at any time, even in situations where exercise may be impossible or inappropriate. You can make good use of time during those long car rides in rush hour or at dreary social events by imagining yourself going through the phases of your limbering exercises, or soaring through the air as you ski jump.

Besides being a form of exercise practice, visualization can be used to encourage healing from injury, sickness or imbalance. A simple and effective technique is to study anatomical drawings of the body part in need of healing. Then close your eyes, relax your breathing and visualize that part of your body transforming itself into healthy condition. As you develop the imagery, you may be surprised to find yourself imagining pictures of the body part undergoing changes, or seeing other kinds of imagery which give a symbolic message about the root of your problem or the pathway to improvement. Over a period of time, you'll notice changes in the imagery, until you one day find your organ or body part mended. You can use this technique for prevention as well as healing.

Magda Proskauer, the San Francisco therapist interviewed in the previous chapter, uses visualization as an integral part of her work. She encourages her students and clients to pay attention to the images in their dreams and waking visions, and to incorporate imagery into their body movements during her classes. Dreams and visions are messages from our unconscious and, therefore, doorways to normally inaccessible depths of our psyches. Several of Magda's exercises which focus on the back and related body imagery are included in this section. If you can 'see' a body part, you can feel it better. Once you have experienced the visualization exercises you may use the basic method to invent your own exercises for any body part or condition.

## THE BASIC BREATH

\* \* \*

**All things share the breath.**
Chief Sealth, Duwamish Tribe, 1885

\* \* \*

There are different Proskauer exercises for each part of the body, but the same three-part breath is used in all of them. This breathing cycle is designed to trigger your own natural rhythm gradually. By using this cycle you can let go of imposed rhythms and allow your own to surface. All these visualization exercises use the breathing pattern described as follows.

Lie on your back on the floor. Relax your arms at your sides and let your feet fall out. Close your eyes and feel the way you are lying on the floor. Notice whether any part of your body feels a bit tense or doesn't seem to be resting comfortably on the floor. Now move your focus inside your body and notice where you feel movement as you breathe.

If you feel tense anywhere try imagining that you can breathe into the tension, as though you could actually exhale through that body part. Imagine the breath relaxing your sore muscle as it moves through it. *Breathing into a body part*

is something you can do anywhere, any time you feel tense or nervous. Locate the tight place and 'breathe into it.' The process is remarkably relaxing and can change the whole quality of your movement. Breathe in sync with the tensing (inhale) and relaxing (exhale) of your movement.

As you are doing this exercise loosen your clothing if it is tight at the waist. Let the muscles of your stomach and abdomen relax and let your breath sink lower in your body. Place your hand palm down at the lowest place on your torso where you can feel the motion of your breathing. Let your hand rest on this place awhile, until you begin to feel the rise and fall of your body under your palm from your breathing. Now let your hand and arm relax at your side again. If you see any pictures of yourself or other images during the breathing exercise, remember them and draw or write them down later.

Relax your jaw and open your mouth a little so that you can exhale through your mouth. You

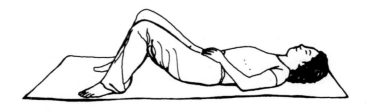

don't need to breathe heavily. Relax and breathe naturally. Inhale through your nose; exhale through your mouth; and pause at the end of the exhalation before you breathe in again.

This pause is the key to the effectiveness of the breathing. Crucial things are happening to your body during the pause; you are still actually exhaling though you may feel as though nothing is going on. Deepening your exhalation gets all the stale air out of your lungs, and makes more room for fresh air when you inhale. Most of us don't exhale deeply enough. Often, when you feel that you can't take in enough air, and that you'd like to inhale more deeply, it's because you haven't exhaled fully enough to make room in your lungs for new air. This is usually the breathing difficulty in asthma. Lengthening your exhalation can help release asthmatic symptoms.

You have paused at the end of the exhalation for a long time now. Let yourself really explore the pause. How does it feel to you? Does it feel too long? Not long enough? Are you a little worried that your body won't breathe in again unless you make it? Think of your breathing when you are asleep. You don't have to tell yourself to breathe then. Think of animals breathing when they are resting. Their breath is long and rolling. They don't tell themselves to breathe. You can learn to trust that your breath will always come in again.

Allow the pause to be as long as it wants. It may feel very long. See whether you can wait and stay with the pause until your body wants to breathe in again by itself. Inhale through your nose; exhale through your mouth; then pause and wait. It's a little like standing on the beach and waiting for another wave to come in. Try to find a pace at which you are neither forcing the pause nor making yourself breathe. Let yourself breathe in this pattern as long as you want.

This exercise in itself is deeply relaxing. If you have difficulty going to sleep you can use this breath at night. Or anytime you feel tense you can take a few minutes off for yourself, relax and find your center again. It is a gentle, powerful centering exercise.

# IMAGE AND BODY MOVEMENT

## The Sacrum

If we can visualize a body part then we can usually feel it better. In order to help keep in balance and to become more sensitive to our backs' functioning, we can visualize our body parts as we move. We can also use other kinds of imagery to develop a sensitivity to body areas that are normally out of sight as the back is.

Magda Proskauer has developed a system of movement alignment which combines breath awareness and visualization. Basic to the visualization in these exercises are the ideas of 'breathing into a body part' and of 'imagining how your joints and muscles look from the inside' as you move. Many of Magda's exercises involve imagining that you can breathe into your pelvis and sacrum, because the nerves and muscles of the sacrum are a major point of release for tension all over the body, especially the back.

To begin this exercise, lie down on your back on a rug or mat. Can you feel your sacrum against the floor? Does it define a particular shape on the floor? Place your palm on your pubic bone. This bone is opposite the sacrum. The pubic bone, pelvis, and sacrum make a kind of bone girdle to support your lower internal organs. What shape is this room?

Imagine as you inhale that the air moves down through your body into your pelvis, filling up this bowl at the base of your spine. As you exhale, imagine that you can send your breath out through your sacrum, into the floor. This exhaling may give you the sensation that with your breathing you are putting down roots into the ground.

Now bend your legs, and bring your knees up toward your chest. Does this change the shape of your sacrum on the floor? Let your lower back muscles relax as you 'exhale through your sacrum.' Allow the area to become as soft and comfortable as a pillow.

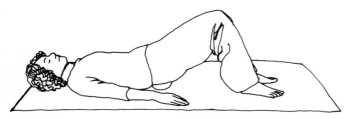

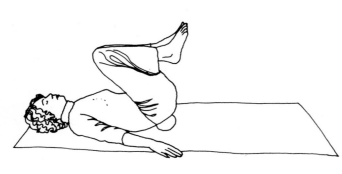

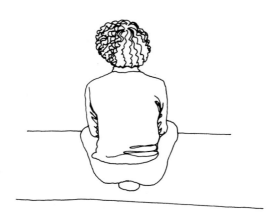

Now place your feet on the floor and press down, raising your sacrum slightly off the ground as you do. Take a small rubber ball and place it under your sacrum in a comfortable place. Draw your knees up toward your chest again and find a place of balance for your legs. Let your lower back respond to the change of position that results from lying on the ball. Let your shoulders relax on the floor, and hang away from your ears. Allow your hips to relax and hang suspended on the ball. Continue breathing into the space between the pubic bone and sacrum, and now exhale through your sacrum into the ball. Continue this cycle for several minutes.

Now lower your feet to the floor, raise your pelvis slightly, and remove the ball. Gently lower your back to the ground. Do you feel any change in the way that your lower back is resting on the floor? Does your sacrum seem to have a different shape? Does your body feel tilted on the ground? If so, which feels higher, your lower back or your head?

Now sit up slowly, feeling the way your pelvis rests on the floor as you sit. Raise your body slightly off the ground with one hand, and place the ball under your sacrum with the other so you are sitting on the ball. Relax and find a comfortable position. Let your breath fill your pelvis as you inhale. As you exhale imagine your breath flowing down your spine through the ball and into the floor. Do this several times. Then remove the ball and lower your pelvis to the floor. As you sit now, does the space between your 'sit bones' feel any different on the floor? Do you feel a change in the angle of your back and the position of your spine over your pelvis?

## The Spine

If you have a healthy spine, this exercise helps you release tension in your back muscles and experience the relationship of the movement of your limbs to your spinal alignment. It should not be done by anyone with acute back pain.

Kneel on the floor on a rug or mat. Lean forward. Touch your forehead to the ground, and relax your arms at your sides behind you, palms up.

As you inhale, raise your right shoulder up toward the ceiling slightly. Imagine it is your breath that is doing the lifting. Feel your right shoulder blade move in toward your spine as it rises.

As you lower your shoulder, imagine that you can exhale through a spot on your spine between your two shoulder blades. Use your breathing to keep your muscles relaxed and your movements smooth. As you exhale and lower your shoulder, let it fall toward the floor. Now try this movement with your left shoulder. Shift the position of your head from time to time, even resting it to one side, to avoid getting a stiff neck.

Now try the movement and breathing while raising both your shoulders simultaneously. As you lower them, release any tension in your upper back muscles and see how wide you can let the area between your shoulder blades become.

Now roll over onto your side, and then onto your back on the floor. Rest awhile.

Imagine that as you breathe you can exhale down the length of your spine. Imagine your breathing passing through the center of each vertebra as you exhale, relaxing all the nerves and muscles along your back.

Lying on your back, take a rounded, straight stick (a de-broomed broomstick will do) and place it under your spine. Lie down on the broomstick and see if you can relax your muscles enough to even out the pressure along your spine. The position should become comfortable. If you feel too much pressure on any point along your spine, 'exhale' through that vertebra to relax the area.

After breathing comfortably in this position take the stick out from under your back and lie down again. Notice any changes you might feel in the way your back is lying on the floor and in the way any parts of your body make contact with the ground.

When you stand up after doing this exercise, experiment with movements of your arms and legs. Notice how the movement of your limbs feels as though it originates from sections of your spine. Try to keep this awareness as you move throughout the day.

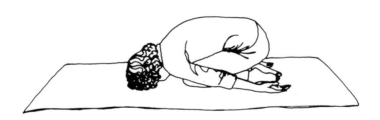

# III
# Special Backs

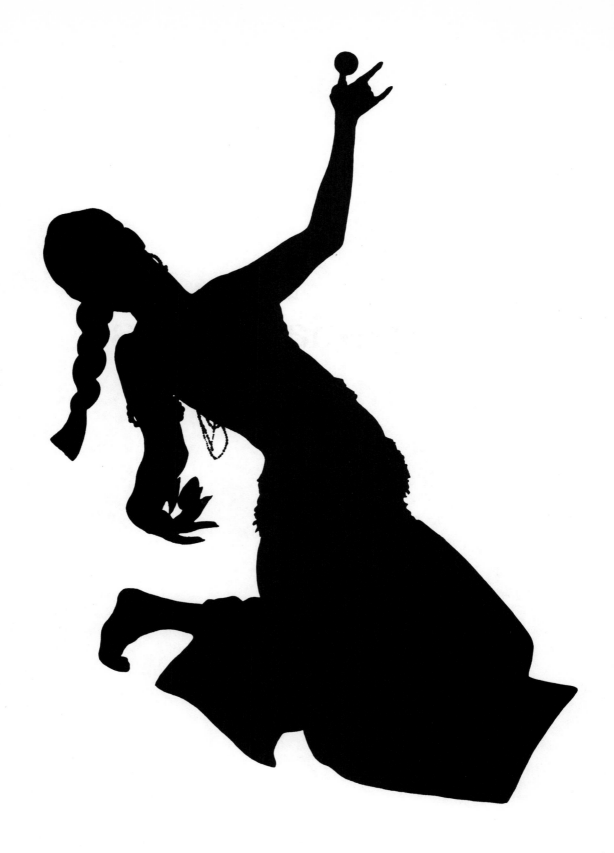

# Pregnancy & Belly Dance: Jamie Miller

Jamie Miller began performing professionally in the summer of 1963 as a member of the San Francisco Mime Troupe. She has been performing as a belly dancer under the stage name 'Sabah' for fourteen years and has helped to reestablish this ancient dance form as an exquisite art. She has taught yoga, creative movement, belly dancing, modern dance technique, improvisation, and experimental acting. In the past two years she has created, performed and produced 'The Erotic Suite,' an original solo piece and is currently in the process of creating 'The Goddess Suite,' her next solo work. Miller lives in Oakland and teaches classes through Berkeley Moving Arts.

## Pregnancy and the Back

I started teaching special classes in belly dancing for pregnant women because the origins of the dance are in birth ritual, and to do this dance with people who are experiencing pregnancy is appropriate, inspiring work. I think that the movements of belly dance originated as a way for women to strengthen their muscles in order to have healthy childbirth. I have a feeling that women also did the movements after they had children to regain good health. If we were all more tuned in to our bodies we would discover these movements naturally. But because we've been in a culture where we're not sensitive to our bodies, we have to take classes for things which people in another culture might just let themselves experience.

Belly dancing is celebratory, and the process of giving birth should be a celebration. People should feel as good as they can about themselves while they're pregnant. This will help the birth, and help the baby feel good about her or himself. The dance movements are sensual; they feel so enjoyable that if you can do them when you're pregnant, it will give you a whole and positive feeling about yourself and your pregnancy. I see pregnant women change their sense of their bodies through taking my class. I think especially of two women who studied with me from the beginning of their pregnancies until they had their babies. One of the women told me that my class had helped her much more than any of the natural childbirth classes she'd been taking. This was her second child. She had already had a healthy and successful first natural childbirth. It wasn't that she had a prior traumatic experience. I have a feeling that her success must have had a lot to do with the depth of the work. The class has to do with deep body awareness and body acceptance. To be able to feel sensual about your body during pregnancy is important. Natural childbirth classes focus on health, but they're not as sensual as belly dancing. One of the women in the class did a performance for us about a week before she had her baby. This was a powerful experience for me. In a certain sense I felt that I experienced belly dancing for the first time as I watched her. It was like seeing the baby rocked in its cradle. As I danced after her, I felt I understood the spiritual pregnancy of the dance.

What I do in the class with pregnant women is different than what I would do with people who aren't pregnant. During pregnancy you have to be more careful of the lower back. In any belly dancing you have to be careful of the lower back because the movements of belly dancing can be extreme. You have to keep working with people to help them experience the front of their spines and the front of their pelvises. It's common for people to try to hold themselves up by their lower backs. Many Western dance forms, such as ballet, tend to teach that the lower back is the center of energy in the body. So I'm always working with people to bring their consciousness to the front of the pelvis.

I also work a lot with stimulating the action of the psoas muscles, which are the longest and strongest pair of muscles in the body, moving from the front of the pelvis to the spine. These are the muscles that developed when we went from being four-legged to two-legged animals. They form a bridge between the spine, the pelvis, and the thigh bones. Any deeply integrated human movement will be based on psoas action whether people know that or not. The 'camel-walk,' the major movement in belly dancing, is the undulation of the spine. It is an example of psoas action. I think that's why it's so extraordinarily beautiful, because it comes from deep inside us.

I always work with students to help them feel these muscles. When you're pregnant you have to be careful because you're carrying a big weight, and there is a tendency to strain the lower back. If you give in to the weight, you can hyperextend and strain the lower back. One of the images I use is to sense your energy moving up the front of the spine and releasing down your back. I also use the image of letting the spine grow into a heavy tail; then letting your tail keep hanging down. This helps to release and to lengthen the spine. One of the problems with many postural concepts is that they tend to be very static. In fact, we have to deal with gravity every moment and the body is going through delicate adjustments all the time. A static concept of posture is injurious to people. I emphasize posture as process, alignment as motion. Many people think that posture is something that you assume and then try to hold. In fact, what creates tension is trying to hold. In pregnancy the fetus keeps on growing and the adaptability of your posture is tested. Since the fetus is growing and changing, the woman is constantly having to reexperience her own center. Pregnancy just emphasizes the things that we deal with all the time. We should all do this all the time anyway, but non-pregnant people can get away with being less conscious of it.

## Belly Dancing for Men

It's important that men understand that this body work is as important for them as it is for women. In some sense it's more important because women do have the physical ability to become pregnant and they generally pay more attention to their bodies than men. So I like to try to get men to experience their centers in themselves. I learned belly dance from a man who is a beautiful dancer and I have men in my classes. Some of my best students have been men because when a man decides to take belly dancing, he has to make a very deep decision. Women can come and take it more easily. Of course, those who really go on to pursue the dance make a very deep commitment, but women can come try it out easily. A man has to really think it through because the social pressures are against his taking belly dancing.

It is helpful for all of us human beings to remember our animal origins. We are still animals, but we seem to want to forget. The approach to movement is helped when people go back to their own primal origins in their infancy, their growth and development, and in the development of the whole human race. Many of the images I use are animal images. One of the reasons belly dancing is such a powerful form is that it evolved from the primal level and expresses that level of existence. There is an undeniable power at this level. It can be felt even by people who shy away from it. They may get upset, but they'll still feel it.

## Origins

Belly dance power has to do with being connected to the earth. Much of belly dancing comes from North Africa. The foot and weight and leg movements are connected to the earth. This connects the pelvis with the earth, and the flow of movement energy is toward the earth. In turn, you let the earth support you. The cycle is an interaction and connection between the person and the planet. From that comes your connection to the universe. The arm movements are 'heavenly,' very spiritual. Belly dancing in its most sophisticated form is able to express many levels of existence simultaneously. You rarely see that kind of sophistication in night clubs because their atmosphere is not supportive. The form, however, is capable of that much integration. You can also think of it as a fusion of many cultures because belly dancing comes from the cultural circle around the Mediterranean: Africa, Asia and Europe, another reason why it's such a rich form.

Belly dancing can be extremely important after pregnancy. During pregnancy people should be careful with the abdominal movements because they may be too severe. You wouldn't want to jar the fetus. But after pregnancy, I can't think of anything better for toning abdominal muscles than the movements of belly dancing. I have never seen any other form of movement that tones the torso so deeply and is so good for all the organs. After giving birth it would speed your healing process because belly dance movements send energy into the depth of your body in a way that most forms don't. I change my emphasis in a class of pregnant women because normally I teach dance as a performing art. In all my beginning classes I help people get into themselves, and it really isn't until intermediate or advanced work that I begin to develop the performance aspect. When I'm teaching belly dancing for pregnant women it's more specialized. I don't expect people to be able to move as well when they're pregnant. Most women do feel awkward when they're pregnant. As a teacher, I wouldn't think of demanding the same kind of exertion from students who are pregnant as I do from those who aren't. And pregnant women are dancing for themselves usually, not for an audience.

## The Pelvis

The warm up series that all my students begin with is done mostly on the floor. We start in a sitting position with sit ups and breathing. I work with breathing throughout the whole process. No matter how advanced someone gets, the breath is still one of the primary skills that we're always working on. They learn to let the breath drop into the sit-bones, then the pelvis, then the spine. We breathe to get energy flowing through the spine. I do some beginning work with arms and the whole shoulder area, which is the most complex musculature in the body and the hardest part of the body to teach because your muscles have to be released to move well. The first step is to get people into their pelvis. You can't even begin arm work until your pelvis is relaxed. The more connected you get to the earth, the more you can embrace the heavens. Then we work on releasing the shoulders. This muscle girdle has a lot of connection to the heart chakra. Many of us hold ourselves up by our shoulders. The more you can release the tension in your body, the more you can accept your sexuality and your fears, the more you can love. It's an inseparable cycle.

After beginning arm work, we do yoga postures which release energy to the spine. I work with the students on all fours. This position is particularly good for pregnant women or for people with back problems, because the spine is released and does not have to fight gravity. As soon as you stand gravity compresses your vertebrae. If you have any weakness, either because you're pregnant or because you've injured yourself, you're probably going to go back to your incorrect posture patterns standing up. When you're pregnant, while lying on your back the belly weight presses down on the nerves and on the veins. But on all fours you can work the spine without much pressure.

The skeleton is the framework of the body. Belly dancing is a dance of the flesh.

You really can't belly dance unless you release your muscles. For most Westerners it is strange to be told to let go of their muscles. Most Western dance tends to be hard-edged and focuses on muscles. In belly dancing you release your buttocks. You don't hold your stomach. You can't do belly dancing if you hold yourself rigidly. Belly dancing is a very soft-edged form of movement.

This form of movement says to someone who is pregnant that they can still be beautiful and do the movements even when their stomachs are sticking out. Most Western forms simply do not take into account the fact that a person might be pregnant. They don't seem to have any space for that. You have to quit dancing and that's a terrible thing. As far as I know, belly dancing was originally used in the Middle East and in Africa during childbirth. And I've heard that women belly danced to celebrate and sympathize with the friends giving birth. It is a non-written tradition, so all of us are guessing. But if you go back into your own feelings about what the birth experience is, some kind of understanding is within each one of us. In tribal communities people are closely linked and they share powerfully with each other through their bodies. It makes sense that women would do this for each other.

The stomach roll in belly dance is really a manifestation of the same kind of energy that the womb is going through in the birth contraction. These movements bring to my mind the image of a snake, which is important in belly dancing. We all came into the world through the uterine canal. All of us have experienced the feeling of the rhythmic contraction of the birth canal so within all of us is that knowledge. Belly dancing expresses that kind of knowledge. I often use the image of letting the arms be like snakes for people's arm movements in the dance. And the whole spine should move like a snake.

If you are pregnant you wouldn't be able to do this exercise, but it would be very good otherwise for strengthening anyone's back. You lie down on the floor on your stomach; put your arms down by your sides; pretend that you have no limbs, and see what you can do to move yourself. This forces you to use your psoas muscles and feel them deeply because there are no other muscles to move your torso. We all tend to depend on our limbs too much for movement. This exercise is a good one to try in order to figure out what the psoas muscles feel like, and to strengthen them, and to get a deeper sense of their centers. You learn you don't have to grip with the lower back. The feeling should be always of letting the spine lengthen.

I do a lot of work with the imagery of breathing into the lower back to open up the lower back area, rather than clinching it. This is helpful during pregnancy because the lower back tends to be strained if you're not conscious of your tensions. Whether somebody with a back injury would have the same kind of movement restrictions on them as someone who was pregnant would depend on the extent of their injury. A person with lower back trouble should be very cautious about beginning to move, but they should move. We all have an incredible amount of knowledge within and if you are truly being good to yourself, you will move well. Most of us have been socially trained not to be good to ourselves. Maybe that's the biggest problem.

We can learn from the movements of people from other cultures. You can see in pictures the way that women in Africa and the Caribbean are related to the earth when they move. The "camel walk" is one of the most glorious movments of the spine I've ever experienced. A lot of the beauty of a movement has to do with gravity and accepting gravity, not trying to deny or fight it. The bowl of fruit I carry on my head in my dance called the Fruit Song is a symbol of that gravity, like having a baby in your stomach. The weight of the baby, if you use it properly, helps you stay in tune with yourself. Instead of a burden, what you carry is a gift. That's what body alignment work is about; learning to feel your body as a gift, rather than as a burden.

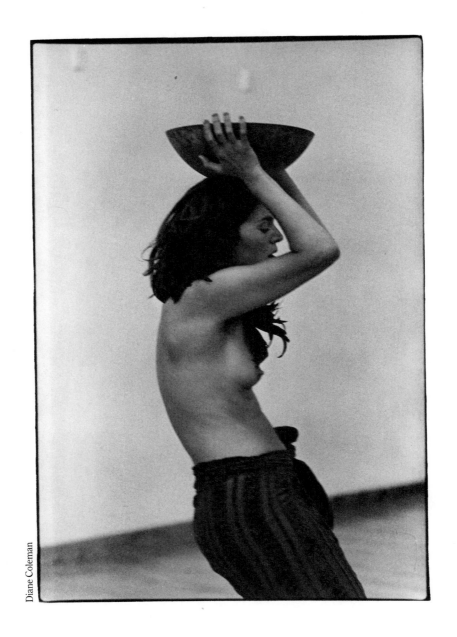

Diane Coleman

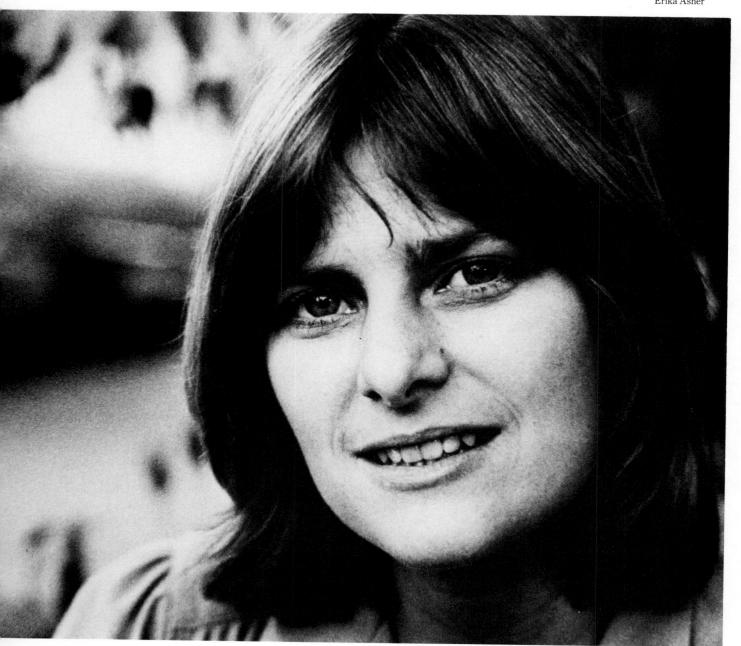

Meg Stern

# Women's Backs: Meg M. Stern

Meg M. Stern began her training in bodywork in 1973 with Maggie Lettvin, a teacher of self-designed fitness courses at the Massachusetts Institute of Technology in Cambridge. Meg set up a low back program for Harvard Medical School in Boston and taught Low Back classes and Fitness For Living classes at Harvard University and Massachusetts Institute of Technology. Meg Stern has combined Lettvin's work with her own methods of postural alignment and tension release. She now teaches individual and group classes in Marin County and San Francisco. Many doctors recommend her classes for their clients and she has worked with doctors on their own spine problems as well. Meg has also done special back alignment classes for the San Francisco Zen Center's Tassajara Bakery Staff whose zazen practice is a challenge to the balance of any spine. Her Zen students report that their back problems have virtually disappeared since their work with Meg. Her work is officially endorsed by both the Lamaze and Bradley childbirth associations.

## Health and Movement

I think the key factors in life which keep people healthy are good nutrition, full breathing and relaxed movements. Moving well is essential. I don't think people can be healthy if they don't move. And we all have to listen to what our bodies tell us and try to accommodate them in our living. This is what I have learned from all my experiences and from my teachers.

Maggie Lettvin, my teacher at M.I.T., was in a car accident. She suffered a slipped disc, a dislocated shoulder, a pinched sciatic nerve and she ended up in a neck brace, unable to move. Instead of having surgery she decided to work on herself. She studied physiology, anatomy, and kinesiology textbooks for information on body movement, and healed herself; it took her two years. Before the accident Maggie ate junk food, smoked, and didn't exercise. After the experience of healing herself she was moved to teach her exercise program to other people through M.I.T.

One of the side effects of exercising is that I feel depressed less often. When I'm lazy on vacations I notice I feel sluggish, have less energy and lack the discipline that I have when I'm exercising. These discoveries spurred me to explore ways of moving which increase psychological and physical health.

The "Fitness for Living" exercise classes I teach now stress postural alignment as a key to fitness and good health. In a non-competitive group we work to increase strength, stamina, endurance, and to gain flexibility while improving the shape and health of our bodies. Each hour begins with an aerobic workout—exercises to improve circulation and respiration in order to strengthen the heart. The rest of the hour is spent exercising specific areas: upper back, hips and thighs, belly muscles, neck and shoulders. By improving muscle tone and posture, weight is redistributed as you develop a strong and healthy body.

By understanding how muscles work, people learn to exercise more efficiently in order to achieve greater strength and flexibility. Without flexibility we feel stiff and lose the muscle tone necessary to support our body weight. Also our muscles must be strong in order to protect our joints from too much stress. My classes provide a balance between working muscles to make them long and strong as well as supple and flexible. I don't think we have to associate getting older with having aches and pains. We aren't in any way destined to be crippled or arthritic, if we take the time to exercise now. And it's never too late to start moving. A natural part of our aging process is that the tissues around joints and muscles lose their elasticity. To maintain normal muscle function and joint movement we must exercise to prevent the loss of elasticity and response in muscles, joints, and ligaments, which would dictate a less functional lifestyle. Participating in a regular exercise program makes you feel better, look better, and helps to relieve such things as headaches, varicose veins, pot bellies, low energy levels and fat accumulation.

In my classes for back and neck problems I focus on back treatment but I treat the whole body, as you must, to heal any one part. My classes are open to people at all levels of fitness and everyone works at their own pace. I do not diagnose. It doesn't matter what the cause of a physical problem is. When you have a headache, you have a headache whether it came because you got hit over the head or because you had a bad day at the office. The important focus is, now, what are we going to do about it? Many people, especially women, are told, "It's just stress" or "It's just in your head." I think that's foolish. It's in their bodies. You can see that. And working through the body and leaving their heads makes them less self-conscious. I never say to them, "Connect your feelings when you're breathing." It happens. You can't separate them. But I don't emphasize the emotions. Especially since taking care of our bodies, i.e., allowing for good feelings, pleasure and hopefully the absence of pain and distress is considered indulgent or a waste of time by so many people.

The process of discovery really has to come from yourself. In order for any self-healing process to work you have to be committed to taking care of your body, and you can't expect that your teacher or some other person will care for it for you. The healing has to become a part of your daily routine. A person has to be committed on a day-to-day basis to moving and breathing correctly. The healing won't work if you put yourself on hold between classes.

## Menstrual Cramps and Pregnancy

Working with women, I find that those who have severe menstrual cramps often have very stiff lower backs and they can barely move the pelvic region. When they start relaxing the pelvic area their cramps often go away. If you have menstrual cramps, you can do the regular, lower back exercises to prevent them. For example, if you get your period on the thirtieth of the month you should start exercising at the beginning of the month and you probably won't experience cramps to the same degree, if at all.

The key is prevention. I see pregnancy as just another type of stress that we have on our bodies. It's foolish not to take the time to take care of your body before you get pregnant. But even if you haven't, you don't have to endure all the discomforts that have become associated with pregnancy. You can start taking care of your body and exercising as soon as you know you're pregnant. You can only expect your body to perform well for you under stress if you do something special to help it.

I recommend doing pelvic floor exercises, or Keigel Exercises; that is, contracting and releasing your vagina and anus muscles fifty or sixty times a day. This can be done any time you urinate by stopping the urination and releasing it several times to strengthen the muscles of the pelvic floor. Because no one can see what you're doing, you can do pelvic floor exercises anytime: when you cross the street, while driving, in a meeting. They don't take extra time; they just take the thought.

If people start to make some accommodations in their daily life, like walking instead of driving as often as possible, that reduces the actual time they need to devote to exercise. It helps your circulation and strengthens your muscles. Or when you're lying down looking at TV, do some exercises. Having a flabby and out of shape body after pregnancy is absolutely uncalled-for. It doesn't have to be.

## Belly Muscles and Your Lower Back

When you're pregnant, as the baby grows and your uterus expands and becomes heavier, pressure is put on your abdominal muscles. It becomes even more important to keep your belly muscles strong and toned so that they will help carry the increasing weight of your baby. And this helps to keep the stretching of your skin to a minimum. Weak abdominal muscles allow your skin to overstretch. Strong belly muscles will help you avoid backaches, keep your stretch marks few or not at all, and will help you enormously as your center of gravity and balance change with your weight change.

During pregnancy all the belly muscles need to be exercised often, to develop the strength needed to support not only the baby but also your spine. As the weight of your baby begins to push your abdomen forward your back moves forward and arches more. The more forward your belly is allowed to hang the more your back will arch. Strong belly muscles prevent your spine from arching too much and help keep your pelvis forward.

Belly muscles are spine supporters. Anyone with even a mild backache is being told by their pain or discomfort that the belly muscles which wrap around their middles and attach along their ribs and along their lower backs are not strong enough to support their body weight.

With the added stress of pregnancy, daily exercising becomes very important. If you do traditional belly exercises, you'll develop overstretched or elongated belly muscles. You have to work at either end of the muscles, not do full sit ups once your belly looks big. Otherwise after you have the child, the muscles will be so stretched that you will need to work harder to recover normal belly tone after delivery. You also don't want your rectus to bulge. These are the muscles down the midline of the abdomen. On weight lifters or body builders, you can often see the separation of the rectus muscles. When you're pregnant and the fetus is stretching the belly muscles, you don't want to increase the stress line by doing strenuous belly exercises.

Instead you should work on developing your side belly muscles, the ones that pull your ribs in, the ones that expand to make room for the baby. These muscles come off your ribs in the front and back and then attach in the pelvis around your crotch and your groin. As more stress is put on the front of your belly, you need to exercise the side muscles so that you don't bulge in the middle. Since your ribs expand to make room for the baby as it comes up, the rib muscles are stretched. You need to strengthen them so your rib cage won't stay stretched out after delivery. I've seen a lot of women whose ribs have come out during pregnancy and won't go back in again. That's because they haven't developed their belly muscles enough during pregnancy and after the baby's born.

You can bring your ribs back in by working the muscles that pull them in. You do this with breathing and with exercise. When you're pregnant your weight comes forward as the baby grows and the muscles are being pulled forward in your lower back. This increases the arch in your back. In order to keep your pelvis forward and to decrease the arch in the lower back, you must have strong belly muscles and pelvic floor muscles to hold you in place. The weight of the baby in the enlarging uterus presses down and the only support for the uterus is the pelvic floor. If you don't exercise the pelvic floor along with the belly muscles, you start to sag. That allows your uterus, your bladder, and your colon all to shift forward slightly, enough to give you problems in pregnancy and after. Too much unsupported weight pressing on the pelvic floor cuts off the circulation in your legs and can cause swollen ankles, muscle cramps, fatigue, and the sensation that you need to urinate frequently.

There are distinct stages for exercises during different stages of pregnancy. In the beginning I work a lot on getting people to walk in place, and later to jog in place. The main artery to the diaphragm that goes into your limbs is pressured constantly when we're pregnant. If we don't breathe well and exercise our legs, the pressure builds up and that's one of the things that allows varicose veins to develop in our legs. Hemorrhoids are varicose veins caused by too much pressure on the colon. There is less chance for these problems to develop by exercising to keep those muscles toned. What particular exercises you should do depend on the size of your belly. Everybody grows differently but the big change is usually around the fifth or sixth month. Then you should not come to a full sit up; just do partial ones.

## Breathing and Childbirth

My work has been endorsed by two natural childbirth associations as enhancing their techniques. The Lamaze technique has you breathe in your chest and your ribs. The idea is to use the breathing techniques as a form of distraction. It works well for some people. Bradley technique teaches you to breathe deeply with your diaphragm and to go with each contraction, to be absolutely aware of the sensation, to go with it on every breath. You're encouraged to breathe fully and deeply and for the few seconds when it's stressful, it *is* stressful, but you breathe deeply which helps you to relax deeply. This really aids in second-stage labor when the baby's coming down and you have to push and to move. Everything functions much better when you breathe that way because you're using all your lower belly muscles. This keeps your pelvis forward and your back flatter while relaxing the pelvic floor muscles at the same time.

Both processes are important alternatives to traditional medically directed labor and delivery where the woman has less control over the birth of her baby. Natural delivery is also a much more difficult process because you are in touch with everything that is happening and you know that sometimes it may hurt. But you do go at your own pace and you work *with* your muscles rather than against them. Also with Bradley when you are "breathing your baby out," you will not breathe it out until your vagina is stretched and open enough to have the baby come through. This means you don't usually have to have your perineum cut which weakens the muscle terribly.

The hospital position, on a table with feet up in stirrups, is not correct for childbirth. To ask a woman to be in that position is torture. You should be able to walk. If you can breathe and walk while in labor you're way ahead of the game. And if you've been practicing and exercising, you *can* breathe and walk. Then for the delivery squat, go on your side, go on all fours or sit leaning back with your legs lying comfortably apart. To have your baby like that is so much better for you and for the baby. In these positions your pelvis is forward; your body isn't pinched and your uterus is in line with your vagina as the baby comes out.

To prepare for an active childbirth you need to do back and pelvic exercises during pregnancy at least, if not before. Some people are so out of touch with their whole pelvic area that they don't know even how to tighten their pelvic floor or move their hips. This cultural inhibition contributes to backaches. If your lower back is stiff, that's an invitation to back problems. In my classes I tease people and say, "Oh, come on, don't tell me you can't move your hips!'' And I may ask them to pretend to write their names with their right hips to make the exercise sort of funny which relaxes people. They say, "Oh, I have a short name, so I'm done first. But Elizabeth really has to work at it!''

If people come to class and stick with the exercises they find that their initial problems pass and they get greater rewards than they had expected. They feel better all the time. They're not so tired. They have new energy. Insomnia, headaches, and many of the tension related symptoms disappear. Many "female" problems disappear with exercise. We stop being the victims of aspirin and girdles. I hope we'll eventually be taught to take care of our whole bodies, just as we're taught to take care of our teeth each day; then it won't be such an enormous task in front of us all the time.

People come to my classes and do the exercises initially because of back problems, but the exercises give you a complete new body image. You become more comfortable with yourself when you move more comfortably. You begin to feel it's o.k. to have this body and not to hate it. It happens for me, and I see it happen with a lot of other people. You start loving your body more when it performs well for you. It's not so important if you don't have those long stereotyped skinny legs and a narrow torso; you start to like your particular body better because it moves for you; it does things for you; it doesn't cause you stress all the time. This attitude is a big payoff, a reward for moving.

Besides a back class, I teach a regular exercise class that's for "healthy" people, which is incredibly exciting to me. Afterward everybody feels so much better. I don't think many of us really experience the health of a well-conditioned body. What we think of as healthy is hardly the beginning of health. We can all feel so much better.

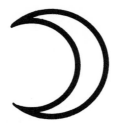

## EXERCISE FOR MENSTRUAL CRAMPS

Besides pelvic breath relaxation (page 96), heat pads, hot tubs, plenty of rest, massage, balanced vitamins and minerals, swimming, and good posture, certain exercises in this book are particularly good for releasing premenstrual lower back tension and menstrual cramps:
The Pelvic Tilt (p. 68)
Salute to the Sun (p. 70)
The Fish (p. 73)
Neck and Spine Stretch (p. 74)
The Cow-Cat (p. 223)
Shiatsu on the Sacrum (p. 143)
Rests (p. 222)

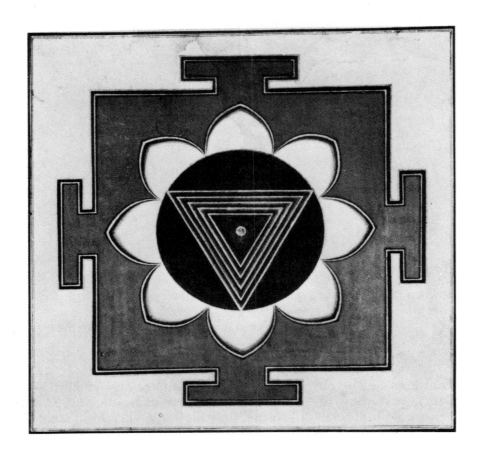

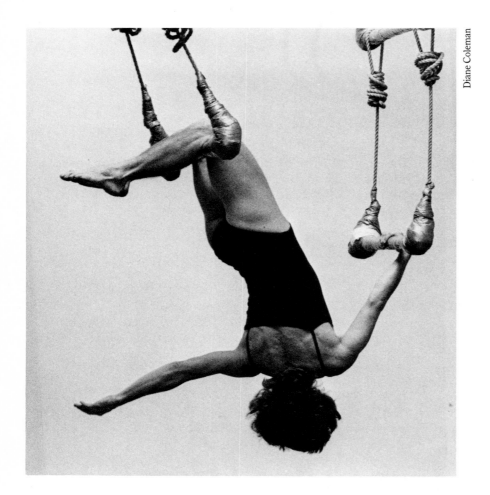

Beyond the diagnosis, the most important treatment of back ache has always been, short of surgery, a therapeutic exercise program initiated once the pain has been controlled. [15]

—Dr. James Nichols, physician to the New York Jets

The mathematician or any citizens whose thoughts are absorbed in some intellectual pursuit, must allow their bodies to have due exercise, and practice gymnastic; and those who are careful to fashion the body, should in turn impart to the soul its proper motions, and should cultivate music and all philosophy.

—Plato, THE REPUBLIC

# The Athlete's Back:
# Martin Kushner, M.D.

Dr. Martin Kushner has been engaged in the private practice of medicine in Seattle, Washington for over fifteen years. Board certified in internal medicine, Dr. Kushner has developed a special interest in the treatment of the muscular skeletal systems, as a result of having worked with many professional athletes.

In my practice I see all kinds of patients. For the most part, I have taken care of three professional sports teams. One is an NBA basketball team; one is a North American Soccer League professional soccer team; and one a World Tennis Team professional tennis team. As a result of this, and the subsequent publicity that one receives from working with professional athletes, I have seen many people who have had various musculo-skeletal complaints. I have taken care of hundreds of people who have had neck and back injuries in automobile accidents. I have also consulted on many cases of musculo-skeletal system injuries for high school and college athletes. I became interested in this work, actually, on a fluke. A good friend of mine was a professional basketball player who had become extremely lethargic and was unable to do his work and unfortunately the team doctor really didn't take enough interest in him, so he came to see me. It turned out that he was severely anemic. I was able, fortunately, to take care of his problem, and consequently a number of the other players on his team came to see me with their various problems. I was subsequently asked to become the official team physician. This was eight years ago, and I have been involved in sports medicine since that time.

## Sport Related Injury

Professional athletes and those involved in heavy sports tend to develop consistent physical problems. Some sports are likely to cause certain kinds of physical problems. In basketball, ankle and knee injuries are the most common injuries which we deal with, other than bumps and bruises. In soccer, our common injuries are knee injuries and pulls of the groin and hamstring muscles. And in tennis most of the problems have to do with the shoulder, elbow, and wrists.

Professional athletes do not seem to have a particularly high incidence of back problems and when they do the problems tend to be relatively minor. The reason for this is that generally athletes know how to take care of their backs and I'm convinced this is the reason that there is a relatively low incidence of back problems. As a general rule, by the time a person becomes involved in professional athletics those back problems which are seen as a result of congenital spondylolisthesis are not present because these people are weeded out early in their athletic careers. This selection process would be true of those people who have back problems as a result of spinabifida. The back problems which I have seen in professional athletes have come from injuries which are sustained in falls and direct blows to the back. Because of the good rehabilitation which is available to them and their generally high motivation factors, these injuries are rather quickly overcome. The traditional medical treatment of sports injured backs is first and foremost rest, until the acute injury subsides. This is followed by exercises, which first cause the back to stretch, and second to build up the abdominal muscles. In addition, during the time that they are resting their backs, we use ice for perhaps the first four to five days, followed by heat and whirlpool. Some people have also recommended ultrasound, but I have found this to be of extremely limited value.

The preventive measures which athletes take to avoid a classical back problem have largely to do with the fact that they are usually extremely well conditioned and also extremely limber. This is less true of football players who tend to get the majority of the back injuries, but these days even football players are working at limbering exercises. We recommend during all sports training, lots of back stretching exercises and having the players avoid those exercises, particularly with weights, which cause the back muscles to flex and decrease the limberness. In addition we recommend exercises to increase abdominal tone, specifically sit up and leg raises. As a general rule among the nonprofessional athletic population, women have more back problems than men do. My experience among professional athletes is that women professional athletes have even fewer back problems than men. I think this is because generally women athletes are even better than men in being limber. And women athletes seem to be extremely well motivated to keep themselves very fit and to have a good strong abdominal musculature.

## Running

Runners, of course, have their own separate set of back problems, which are the result of the constant pounding that the disc spaces take in long distance running. Many runners eventually have to give up running because of this problem despite adequate flexibility and strength. I'm not sure there's an answer to that particular problem, although I have seen several people who, when it was discovered that they had shortening of one leg, and put a heel lift into that shoe, their runner's back problem subsided. This is a particular problem which I don't think occurs as frequently as some other people do, but I think that any runner who finds that they have back problems should definitely have their lower limb length checked to see if a heel lift is necessary. I have also seen runners whose back pain has subsided, either by changing their stride, or mostly by shortening their stride or changing from a toe strike to a heel strike. I'm not exactly sure why these things have helped, but occasionally they do. I think a runner who has been having problems with the back should have another runner run behind them and critique their method of running. I think that this is perhaps the best way that they can effect some changes which may affect the course of their back pain.

The casual runner or jogger is more likely to have ankle or knee pain, but occasionally they too will get back pain, which can be altered by the use of a proper shoe. Good running shoes should have a wide heel and should be rather springy. Also casual runner's back pain can sometimes be lessened by their running on either grass or cinders or a regular track, rather than on concrete.

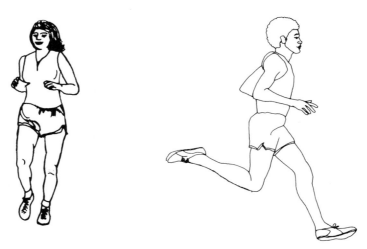

## After Injury

After an injury the first stage of recovery is rest. One should stop the sport altogether after a back injury to allow recovery to begin to take place. With the back one of the major problems becomes muscle spasm, which sets in almost immediately after a back injury and continues when one's sport tends to aggravate this and keep it going for a long period of time. We will stop the athletes from their sport and have them have bed rest for several days. I use anti-inflammatory drugs as well as muscle relaxers. During this rest time, copius amounts of ice are used in packs on the back until the spasm begins to subside and the athlete is comfortable. Following that, we switch to heat treatments and gradual stretching exercises followed by abdominal toning exercises.

I believe that preventive exercise programs are extremely beneficial and my experience has been absolutely that those athletes who take the time to warm up well before they play, whatever their sport is, are the ones who have fewer musculo-skeletal problems. Those whose warm ups largely consist of limbering up exercises clearly have a lower incidence of back problems than those whose do not.

Concerning the question of pain killers, I feel very strongly on this subject. I use pain killers purely as relief for somebody who is in pain and not to enable them to play. I think anybody who engages in professional sports who is hurting enough to require a pain killer is being foolish. And a doctor who recommends pain killers in order to enable people to play is guilty of malpractice. Pain is the body's way of telling us that the injured part needs to be rested and I think the wisest thing one can do under the circumstances is to rest the injured part. Pain killers are, however, necessary when people are experiencing pain, dependent upon their injury, and I see nothing wrong with treating those symptoms.

There are a number of centers of sports medicine around the country, many connected with universities. I'm not sure that it's necessary for an injured athlete to go to one of these sports medicine centers. I think, in general, anyone who has had experience with injuries to athletes can take care of most of the problems which come up.

## Prevention

I'd like to make some general statements about my experience with and feeling about the care of the back in athletes, both professional and amateur. Basically I feel that as we all know, our backs are extremely imperfect structures and were clearly made for us to go about on four legs. One can avoid back problems with proper exercises and proper conditioning. I feel that any athlete first and foremost should be fit. And if they're not fit, they should get fit slowly before thay begin to engage in any heavy athletics. Getting fit entails getting cardiovascular fitness. This causes oxygen to get to the muscles more efficiently. Oxygen is necessary for proper muscle function. Then also the muscle can clear out the lactic acid which eventually builds up, and use oxygen more efficiently. A muscle which is able to do this is less susceptible to injury, and back injuries are largely muscular.

Secondly, once an athlete is fit, each time they engage in any kind of athletic endeavor, they should have the proper warm up and proper cooling down period. This will vary somewhat from one type of activity to another, but should always involve stretching, some warming up and some general toning exercise. This is particularly true in outdoor games in cold weather. The colder the person is and the tighter the muscles are, the longer should be the warm up period. I am of the opinion that anyone who is engaging in athletics should be able to put the full flat of the hand down onto the floor with the knees straight. I've rarely seen anybody who could do this complain of a sore back.

I want to mention one important aspect of rehabilitation. One of the excellent things that one can do in rehabilitating a back after injury once things have subsided somewhat is swimming. Swimming is the exercise par excellence which will help to build up back muscles without any of the pounding which is involved in the running type exercises.

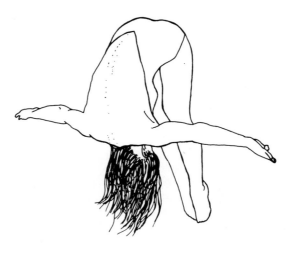

**Everybody in this country now is afraid not of death, but of aging—and of what we've made of the aging process in terms of illness, dependency, and deterioration. So preoccupation with trying to improve that is a reasonable concern.**[16]

—Margaret Mead

**In spring, the orchid, in autumn the chrysanthemum;**
**So shall it be forever, without break.**[17]

—Ancient Songs of Chinese Shamanism

# Life Cycles & Back Again: Adolph Segal, M.D.

Orthopedics is a branch of medicine that seeks remedies for injuries and diseases of bones, joints, muscles, ligaments, and tendons. Dr. Adolph Segal, an orthopedic surgeon, took his formal training at the University of California and was certified by the American Board of Orthopedic Surgery. His medical practice covered the full range of orthopedic problems. He lives in San Anselmo, California, where I visited him to talk about his work. We sat in front of the fire, ate delicious ginger and spinach soup, watched the February rain shaking the forests, and discussed life cycles and healing.

## Orthopedics

In my practice, I worked with a large number of back problems. In the ordinary medical hierarchy orthopedists are generally considered to have the final word for back treatments; back problems make the largest single area of treatment in orthopedics.

I took an eclectic approach to back problems. I would do a complete work-up including a history, a long physical, and x-rays when necessary. Then I would work with the individual in whichever way I felt would be best for him or her.

The conservative management of backs is largely done by orthopedists; surgical management is done by both orthopedists and neurosurgeons. Dealing with the nervous system of the spine is an area in which orthopedic surgeons and neurosurgeons overlap. Some neurosurgeons handle it; some orthopedists also handle it. I didn't particularly like back surgery. Bending over the operating table used to bother my back.

## Structural Evolution

Actually, the back is poorly designed for its functions. Since humans have assumed the upright (orthograde) position, the embryology and structure of the back have been in

Anne Kent Rush

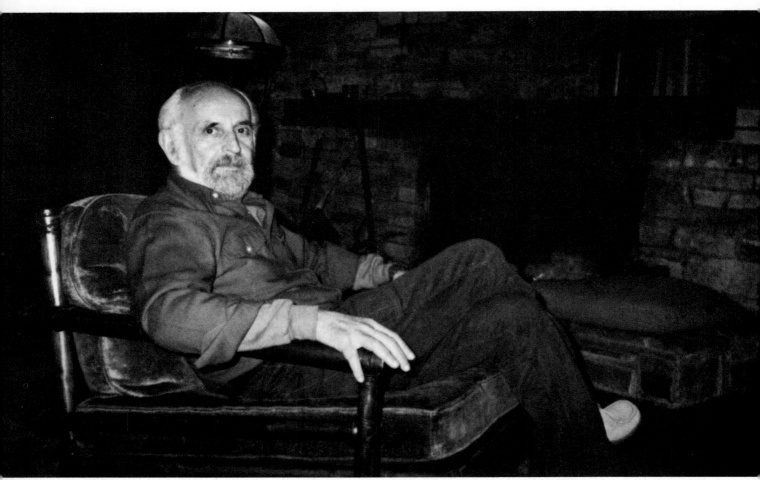

Adolph Segal, M.D.

transition. It wouldn't solve things to return to walking on all fours, of course, because our chests have expanded laterally, and we couldn't get our arms close enough under our bodies to move like animals. Our shoulders have been pushed out sideways, but our hips are still in a rather similar position to those of four legged animals. Standing erect on those structures is not ideal!

Given the way that the sacrum fits onto the pelvis, the lower portion of the spine is not only structurally prone to injury, but it is constantly being traumatized by gravity.

You can't get away from gravity, unless you go to outer space or under sea where you're weightless. Here on earth, gravity will wear on you, even as you sit right now. It's hard on your feet, your legs, your back, your whole structure. The physical effect on the back is that gravity's pressure wears it out. That's often demonstrated by the fact that many people are shorter when they're older than they are at maturity.

## Childhood

At birth, babies' spines are generally straight. As they move more in relation to gravity, as they crawl, sit and walk, they develop the compensatory curves in the spine that allow them to remain upright. The large spinal adjustments come when a baby moves from lying down to sitting up. Generally speaking, if a child has been sitting satisfactorily before starting to walk, she or he will have little spinal change as a result of walking because the spinal mechanics and statics of walking and sitting are essentially similar.

In children, backaches are due to injury by and large. For instance, a child may fall out of a crib or tree and injure the spine, but sprains and strains from, say, lifting, etc., are virtually unknown in children. Backaches in children may also be the result of disease. A child may have a blood stream infection which settles in the vertebrae. Malignancies in children can also cause backaches. Unfortunately child abuse must be included as a cause of children's back problems.

## Teens

With teenagers, profound injury becomes more common because teenagers tend to be more vigorous and violent in their activity. It is at this age, and primarily in female children, that scoliotic curves manifest and these are usually harmless. Teens often pattern their posture after their parents' posture. Much scoliosis is "hereditary" in this sense. Teenage girls often feel emotionally and physiologically in upheaval while adjusting to menstruation. If they have very curved spines, they may opt for pain in the back in order to get attention or avoid problem situations at school or home. Or, worried about appearance, they may think their curve is more of a cosmetic problem than it need be.

I found treating teens from age thirteen to, say, eighteen, difficult. One minute they're adults and the next minute they're infants. And because they're not yet sufficiently trained or developed, the boys often have many sports injuries.

## Twenties and Thirties

Young adults most often suffer spinal sprains and strains. I think at their age, the back becomes the prime target for work-related, and neurotic sex-related malfunctions. These can become tough problems of management. You have to deal not only with the injury, but with a frequently delayed motivation to get well in young working adults. As long as a worker is not recovering, he or she may be receiving unemployment or other compensation. This often conflicts with recovery from the back problem. The statistical difference between the recovery of individuals who are injured at home doing their own schtick and those individuals who are injured in industry is vast. Private patients who have no industrial compensation do infinitely better. They generally get well faster because they are motivated to get back to their shop, or to whatever work they do, since staying disabled brings no financial benefit.

Also in this age group, as women begin having children, back problems related to childbearing develop. The burden of childcare, with its dearth of adult contact, and the changes in sexual attitudes which come about, bring a special kind of isolation and stress. New physical modes like bending over into a crib improperly, bending over to wash the child, or picking up heavy lethargic kids who may be irritating the mothers anyhow can easily lead to the onset of back problems. Young mothers are often tense and this increases their susceptibility to back problems. They may find that a backache can become an escape for getting out of distasteful chores. But if you can get new mothers to talk about the real factors involved, their conditions often clear up when they begin tackling their basic dilemmas at home.

## Forties and Fifties

Technically I think it's correct to say that aging begins at twenty for most people. For the musculo-skeletal system, it's a downhill trip from twenty on, and the signs of this degeneration usually surface in the forties. Usually older individuals show more changes, less range of motion in the joints, less functional capacity, more disability. At late ages you see once again, fairly significant numbers of malignancies, both primary and metastic to the spine. As people pass the age of sixty, degenerative problems of the back such as disc wear, spurs, and arthritis often ensue. "Arthritis" is a catch-all term that often doesn't mean anything specific. It's usually applied to complaints of pain, stiffness, and restricted activity. It's rare for an individual to reach the age of forty or fifty without having had a back problem. And I'm just talking about the lumbar and the sacral areas, eliminating problems of the cervical and thoracic spine.

## Old Age

The best work on the later age phases that I know of is done at the Sage Center in Berkeley, California. They're doing magnificent work with older people, dealing with backaches and stiff joints and many other physical and emotional problems of old age. Among other things the staff at the Sage Center teaches older people a little yoga, some dance, some exercises, and how to massage each other. They get the individual interested in and excited about life. Turning them on to living is often equivalent to turning off their discomfort.

A lot of the people like athletes who exercise heavily and consistently may have more advanced aging changes than the more sedentary types, as a result of prolonged, strenuous physical activity. And psychologically those people may have a self-image which puts high demands on them to perform well physically, no matter what age they are. It's difficult to generalize about what sort of exercise is best for people. Mild exercise may maintain optimum health for some people contrary to the dogma of many physical fitness faddists.

Swimming is good for the back primarily because it's one of the few conditions in which you can get partial release from the stress of gravity and still exercise. Your buoyancy in the water allows you to exercise with less wear and tear.

I don't think there is any universal panacea. Some people will respond well to one path. Others will be absolutely devastated by it. An eclectic approach to whatever physical activity would be beneficial for the particular individual is best.

## Nutrition

Good nutrition is a significant factor all through life. There are a lot of diet fads, but the answer lies somewhere in between them and junk food. A good deal of our ultimate endurance of wear and tear, and our potential for longevity and peak emotional and cerebral functioning has to do with what we're made of chemically. The body is such an incredible system that it can detoxify most of the unhealthy foods we put into it. But if we "poison" ourselves with chronic malnutrition for forty years or so, we'll manifest health problems. The results of eating poorly may not show up at first but ultimately it taxes the whole organism—body, mind, and spirit. With my patients, I would generally check over their dietary regime, and if it was perfectly obvious that they were eating bacon and eggs every morning, lots of butter, and lots of sugar and cream and they were obese as a result, then I would suggest certain changes that I thought might help.

It's easy to become confused about what good nutrition is. Here in America we theoretically have adequate food, and lots of fresh fruits and vegetables. But we don't know what is in most of them, or what's contaminating most of them. So I have to go a lot by good common sense. Whether we need vitamin supplements or not is an open question. It's too complex; much of the information we have about diet is vastly contradictory. You can find authorities of equal stature on opposite sides of any question. Health food stores can be one of the biggest shucks because their food often isn't really any different. And I frequently see more ill-looking people in health food stores than in regular markets! Rigid dietary fanaticism can be unhealthy too.

## Stress

As far as I can see, stress is probably the greatest single cause of back problems. By stress, I don't mean the ordinary stimulation that we all need to keep functioning. I'm talking about the stress related to living in our society. Stress encompasses almost every cause of back problems, whether it's stress on the system resulting from malnutrition, or stress in relation to society, to sexual problems, to children, or to your inner microcosm. When stress is sufficiently heavy it becomes a factor in producing distress. What individuals are really dealing with is distress, whether it manifests as a backache or as a malignancy. In making a diagnosis you have to be sensitive to the effects of every kind of pressure.

## Healing

My attitudes toward medicine have gone through some distinct stages. I started, in classical fashion, with scientific training, and along the line, was influenced by a number of people. The ideas of Alan Watts affected my philosophy. David Cheek, M.D., an obstetrician and classmate of mine, is a world-renowned practitioner of medical hypnosis. I witnessed his treatment of a brain problem by hypnosis which altered my way of looking at the usual organic medical problem.

Then I saw an anthropologist's film of various fire-walking cults, and that changed my opinions profoundly. In medical school I had learned that protein subjected to heat denatures. But in the feet of these firewalkers, it didn't. This challenged all my thinking. If protein could respond in a fashion unlike anything I had learned, then I had to rethink all my medical training.

This re-examination of science led me to explore Eastern philosophies. The whole business of what health was, and what curing was, came into question. I quit medicine for a while because it was too disturbing to do something and not believe it completely. This was about twenty years ago.

Subsequently, I studied more and more of the so-called unscientific methods of approaching medical problems. I explored hypnosis. Esalen, yoga, biofeedback, autogenic training, acupuncture, Rolfing, polarity therapy, and so on. I took a taste of many kinds of healing. Each discipline failed to make a convert of me. But each had parts that I could use. So my answer became to be more eclectic instead of more specialized. To my own techniques I added whatever techniques were advanced or acted as healing agents. By the time I completely quit operating about five years ago, except for certain difficulties, I had found I could help heal without surgery many problems which I had previously considered to be correctable only through surgery.

## Communication

I finally realized that the most important thing I could do was listen. If I simply sat and gave someone my full, undivided attention for as much time as they needed, they frequently didn't need to come back. I was putting myself out of business! But I think that ultimately this was the most significant thing I got out of all of these various paramedical explorations. The most important thing was communication. People could express their fears and simply feel completely free to say whatever they wanted, and they were often greatly benefited. The simple reassurance that it was o.k. to have what they had was all that was required for a significant number of people. A few needed cortisone, aspirin, physical therapy, etc. But the real changes happened in the communication.

I think it's important to focus on what heals. And it keeps getting back to the fact that the relationship you have, either with the person you're working with, or with yourself, is the most important thing. I don't know what healing is. And I've spent my life as a professional healer. People would say to me, "I got all broken up in an auto accident and you operated on me and put all my bones back together." Well, I can put you back in line. I sew up your skin. But I don't do the healing. The operation doesn't heal the skin. No one knows what's at the core of the process of healing. I know what it looks like microscopically. I know the stages that you go through, but what triggers it?

And what triggers nonhealing is another mystery. You can delve into metaphysics, and the paradoxical logic of Eastern philosophy. But no one can pin it down. There's no one answer, but it's important to figure out a way to communicate in a language that approximates the complex dynamics of healing. That's hard when you're talking medicine, which is supposed to be the one answer.

The fragmentation of healing into many competing disciplines and factions can prevent healing. The body works as a whole. The body and psyche are one functionally. I think we should be happy to use any branch of healing if it works. It can come to much ado about nothing to give techniques specialized names like biofeedback or acupuncture or physical therapy. I am a pragmatist: if it works, it works. None of us knows what the phenomena of the process of healing are.

To heal, we must be open to the entire spectrum of our human experience, and to the unknown aspects which we cannot or have not defined. Even when an individual is exercising well and eating a perfect diet, if his head is confused and upset, his health can be terrible.

Trying to diagnose, you come to a point where strictly metabolic studies are inadequate, because they don't take in the unknowns. And isn't it the unknown that is controlling the machinery?

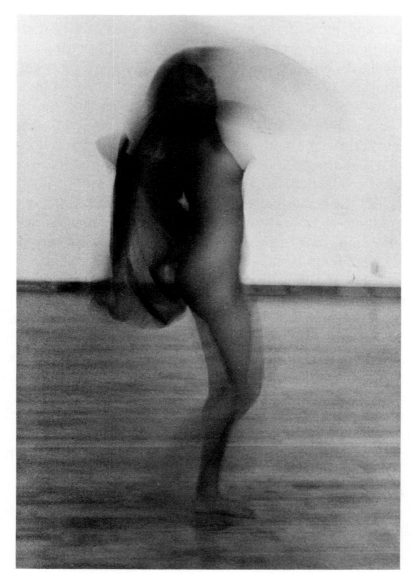

Diane Coleman

132

# IV
# The Sensual Back

# SENSUALITY—SECTION IV: CONTENTS

**On Healing and Pleasure**

**Back Massage:** Preparation; Centering; The Basic Back Stroke; Trapezius Squeeze; Blade Lift; The Middle Back: Rib Map; Side Strokes; The Lower Back: Shiatsu on the Sacrum; For the Buttocks; The Neck: Shiatsu Points; Head Stroke; Whole Spine: Spine Stretch; The Waterfall; Thumb Squeeze; Cross-hatching; Spine Snake; Grand Finale; Room for Creativity; Head to Toe; Centering Energy

**A Dancer on Sensuality: Jamie Miller**

**A Survey**

**Sex and Backaches:** Positions After Injury; Sit Ups; Staying on Top of It; Injury Positions; Spoons; Half Sit Up; Let Rest; Profiles; Face to Face; Neck Pain During Sex; Strengthening the Pelvic Floor; Massage, Saunas, Jacuzzi

# On Healing & Pleasure

Our ideas and experiences of pleasure affect how we decide to take care of our bodies. Everyone has a personal pleasure quota, a limit on how much pleasure he or she can experience. We are attracted to other people who share our sense of proportion for work and play, for asceticism and hedonism. Most of us could benefit from increasing our pleasure quotas by quite a few degrees.

Living in our fast paced, industrial world, we are caught up in the impetus to meet deadlines in spite of our strained emotions, to keep schedules unfit for our bodies' rhythms, to work in inhuman environments. Few of us choose to flee to the wilderness. If we embrace the nervousness of New York, the hype of L.A., the hustle of Hong Kong or the pressures of Paris, we will have to invent ingenious ways to stay healthy in the urban environment.

We all have the intuitive knowledge to sense what is good for us. But this impulse for self-healing is often counteracted by the attitude that only an outside expert can cure us, and by a lack of faith in the practicality of pleasure. Consequently advancement in the world of work often proceeds in direct proportion to our health's decline. We neglect relaxation in the face of seemingly more important pressures. There is, of course, a need for restraint in our indulgence of egotistic or social hedonism; but on a personal level within our daily routines and our intimate lives there are fruitful realms to explore.

We could let go of the common attitude that places activities which only make us feel good at the bottom of our priority lists. We are rarely encouraged to set aside time from our daily chores to renew ourselves in mind and body. Yet if we do not take time to balance pleasurable activities with compulsory ones we risk becoming physically ill and the more subtle damage of being drained of flexibility, spontaneity and creativity.

Most of us feel a little anxious when we consider increasing our pleasure quotas. Do we fear that we'd get less work done? Or that other people would criticize us for being selfish? Does pleasure seem like a realm in which we have less control than in others?

Do we fear our taste for pleasure would run away with us? Do we harbor the philosophy that misery and struggle are more character-building states than pleasure?

No one inherently wants to avoid pleasure except out of fear. The fears connected with experiencing pleasure are best cured by experiencing more pleasure, and discovering that it usually enriches rather than hampers one's life. Soon your quota is raised and a new level of pleasure becomes the norm. You'll find yourself functioning more smoothly with fewer breakdowns and conflicts. One of the best healers for anxiety is pleasure. Go get a massage and think about it.

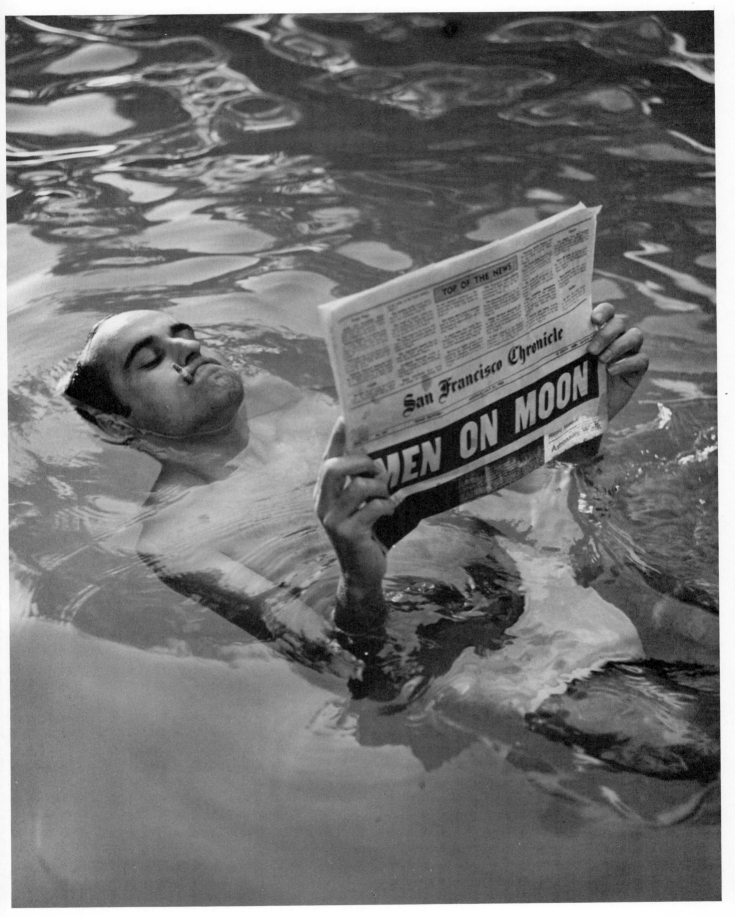

Elisa Bowen

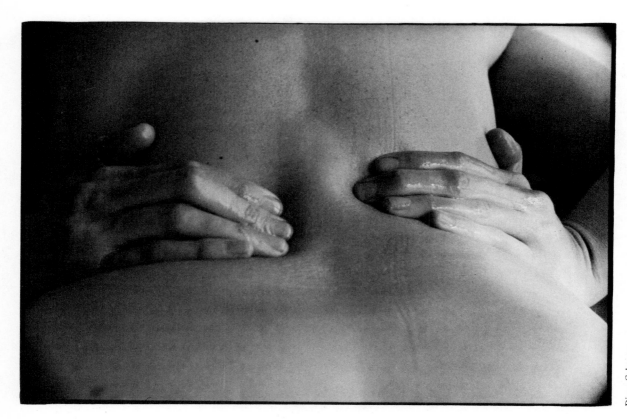

Diane Coleman

# Back Massage

There is no pleasure quite like that of a good back massage. Combining the medical benefits of physical therapy and the comfort of a mother's caring with the stimulation of a sensual treat, the back rub seems to rate high on everybody's list of favorite things. As body therapy, back rubs are soothing because a complex system of nerves radiates from the spinal cord to almost every part of the body and by massaging the back nerves you can relax your whole body. Massage can improve circulation, relax tight muscles, and release rigid connective tissues. You can ease tension throughout the body by relaxing the back. Receiving a back rub is often experienced as a luxury because touching the back can be sensual without being demandingly sexual. And giving can be as pleasurable as receiving as one delves into the lovely planes and valleys of one of the largest expanses of smooth skin and muscle in the human form.

\* \* \*

Editor's note: In this section we have selected pronouns to refer to the recipients of the massage or technique according to the sexes of the people in the illustrations. Although from our point of view pronouns would ideally refer to everyone, there seems to be no easy way to fudge it here by using an ambiguous plural. We hope our readers will edit the exercises in their minds to apply to themselves as desired.

\* \* \*

## Preparation

If you are planning to give a back massage to a friend, there are several things you should do to prepare. Choose a quiet room. A beach towel or sheet will do for your friend to lie on if the surface underneath is smooth and soft, perhaps a rug or a massage table with a foam pad.

If you are standing to give the massage, keep your feet about shoulder width apart on the floor and bend your knees slightly at all times. As you bend over for deep strokes let the weight of your body supply most of the pressure, rather than trying to exert pressure by forcing or pressing. Synchronize your movement with your breathing. If you keep these things in mind, you won't hurt or strain your own back while you are doing the massage and your partner will appreciate the ease and comfort of your motion. Have a bottle of warm massage oil within easy reach.

## Centering

Have your friend lie on his stomach, with his head to the side that is more comfortable. Rest the palms of your hands on his shoulder blades simply to make contact before the massage begins. Take these few moments to close your eyes, relax your breathing, and center your own energy before you begin the massage.

### The Basic Back Stroke

This stroke is very relaxing and covers the whole back, so it is usually a good way to begin.

Take some oil from the bottle beside you, holding the bottle in one hand while keeping your elbow or part of your forearm in contact with your friend's back so that you don't lose touch. Squeeze some oil into your palm; rub your palms together so that you warm the oil before you put it on your friend's back. There are few sensations less appealing than having cold oil poured on you when you are expecting a relaxing massage. Continue to apply the warmed oil until your friend's whole back, from the shoulders down to the top of the thighs, is lightly covered with oil.

Place your palms on either side of your friend's shoulder blades at the very top of his back. Have your fingers pointing toward each other and your elbows out. Lean your body weight down into your friend's shoulders so that your palms are pressing into the back and your fingertips are on either side of the spine. Few massage strokes actually press down on the vertebrae. The strokes are usually most comfortable

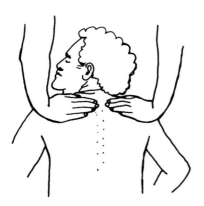

when you are pressing on the muscles on either side of the spine.

Now angle your body weight down and forward, and slide your palms all the way down your friend's back from shoulders down to the waist. Keep your fingertips pressing into the muscle furrows on either side of the spine. As you reach your friend's lower back, keep the pressure firm but begin to separate your hands. Make a half circle with your fingertips, first pointing to the vertebrae and then rotate them outward till they're pointing toward the sides of the table, and your hands end up on either side of your friend's hips.

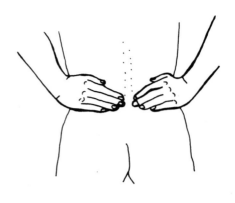

Now your hands are in a position where your palms and fingers are holding your friend's hips. Grasp your friend's hips a little more firmly and use this hold to lift the torso slightly and pull up on the muscles of your friend's sides as you lean back. The next motion of this stroke is done by letting your body weight pull your arms and hands back up all the way from your friend's hips to the shoulders. As your palms pass over the ribs, squeeze with your thumbs and fingertips lightly. This part of the stroke is wonderful to receive because you almost feel that you are being lifted off the table; you can let go of a lot of muscle stress.

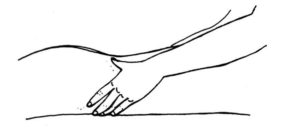

When your palms are resting on the top of your friend's shoulders again, pivot your fingertips so that they are facing each other, and begin the stroke again. This stroke feels best if it continues as a cycle of leaning down and lifting. You can repeat the stroke quite a few times because it is very relaxing.

If you give the massage on the floor it's good to work in a kneeling position because as you lean forward you can raise up on to your knees; and as you lean backward you can sit down on your heels.

### The Trapezius Squeeze

The trapezius muscles reach from the base of your neck across the top of your shoulders. They are usually a firm band of muscles, often quite tight and sore, so they need a lot of attention. When you are standing at one end of the table behind your friend's head, use both hands and squeeze with the thumbs on top and forefingers underneath the shoulders. Use a rhythmic

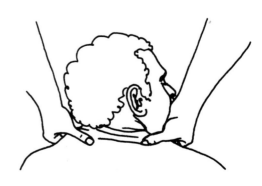

motion to massage the tapezius muscles several times.

Then, pressing your thumbs on top of the trapezius muscles, make small circles all over the area. Use your body weight to lean into the muscles. Cover the whole area of the trapezius muscles with thumb circles, all the way down the neck, across the top of the shoulders, and down the whole area between the shoulder blades.

### Blade Lift

Now have your friend roll on to her side. She should have her head slightly forward with the chin tucked under, the arms relaxed across the chest. The leg lying on the table should be fairly straight, while the upper leg should be bent at the knee to support her. In this position the upper shoulder and shoulder blade are pulled by the weight of gravity toward the table.

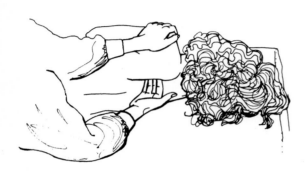

Place the fingertips of your right hand, your palm facing toward you, under the shoulder blade of the person you are massaging. If your friend's muscles are relaxed enough, position your fingertips in between the shoulder blade and your friend's back. The muscles that hold the trapezius to the back often get tight. Massage the muscles in a slow half circle from the top of the shoulder down along the shoulder blade toward the ribs. You can rest your left hand on your friend's shoulder while you are doing this. Then have your friend roll over onto her other side, so you can repeat the same stroke on the other side.

### The Middle Back: The Rib Map

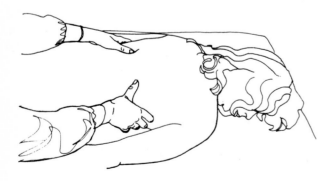

Have your friend roll over onto her stomach again, with her arms relaxed at her sides and her legs relaxed so that the heels are slightly falling out. Use the tips and sides of your thumbs to define the muscles in the space between each rib. Start at the vertebrae between the shoulder blades. Lean your weight slightly into your partner's back. Keep your thumbs on either side of the vertebrae. Slide your thumbs away from each other, defining the area between each rib across your friend's back and down her sides. When you slide your thumbs all the way down to the table, lift your hands and bring them back to either side of the spine. Start on the next rib and work your way down all the ribs.

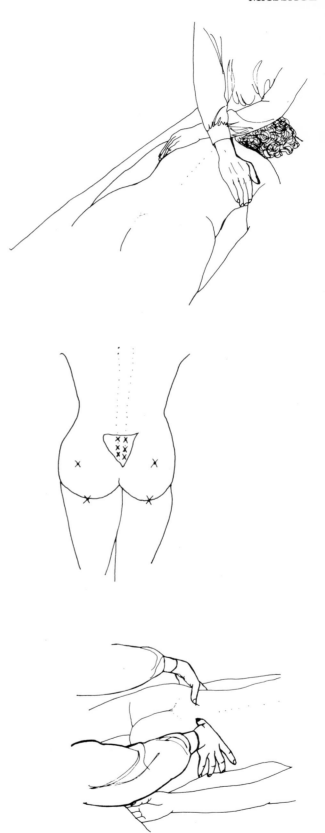

When you reach the last two ribs, lighten your pressure a great deal. Sometimes these are floating ribs which can't bear as much weight as the upper ones. And your partner may be a little ticklish. Using firm pressure will keep this from being a rib-tickling stroke.

## Side Strokes

Use your palms to do side strokes. Begin with the heels of your palms resting on the table to either side of your partner's upper back. Then move your fingertips toward each other, toward the spine. Just before they touch, move your hands slightly away from each other so that they can continue all the way down your partner's sides again to the table.

Now reverse the motion and slide the heels of your hands back to the starting position. Repeat this cross over stroking up and down your partner's back from the shoulders down the back to the hips.

## The Lower Back: Shiatsu on the Sacrum

Shiatsu is a form of pressure point Japanese massage based on the same energy system as acupuncture. Though the complete system requires training, you can use a simple version of pressure point massage for very relaxing effects.

Stand beside your partner's hips. Lean your weight on your arms as you press your thumbs down on either side of your partner's sacral vertebrae. Gradually angle your weight deeper into your hands so that your thumbs are pressing down into the muscles of the sacrum.

When you want to release the pressure do it just as gradually as you applied it, so that your hands come out of your partner's muscles very slowly. Then move your thumbs down to the next sacral vertebrae. Apply the pressure of your body weight again. Work your way from the top of the sacrum to the tip. Then apply the same type of gradual pressure to the lower outsides of the sacrum, from your partner's waist down to the tail bone. The pressure should not be painful in any way to your friend. If it is painful it means you are either pressing too quickly or too hard for her to relax with the pressure. You might not be in quite the right spot, so shift your position and try another spot. Remember that you'll be

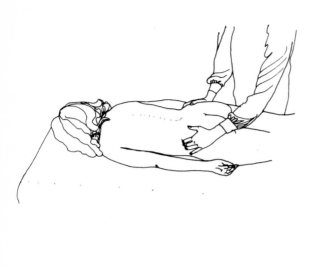

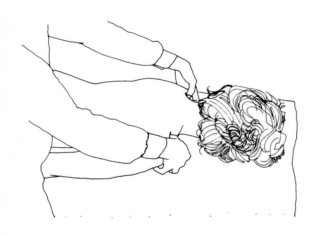

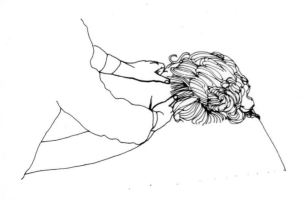

more comfortable if you use your body weight to exert the pressure, rather than just using your arms. This way you should be able to get a great deal of pressure without straining.

## For the Buttocks

The gluteus maximus muscles in the buttocks need lots of massage because they are often quite tense. You can continue the shiatsu all over the hips and buttocks. There are critical acupuncture points in the center of the hips, and there are some relaxation points to press under the buttocks where the thighs join the hips.

Make large circles on the buttocks with the palms of your hands. Stand or kneel just below the level of your partner's hips, resting your body weight on your palms and pressing into your partner's muscles. Slide your hands out and across the hips from the "sitting bones" so that your fingertips make circles over the bones and your palms are massaging the muscles. Next rotate the fingertips out toward the side and bring the heels of your hands back to the beginning position under the "sitting bones" and slightly lift the buttocks. Repeat these strokes several times.

## The Neck: Shiatsu Points

Continue the shiatsu pressure massage. Place your thumbs on both sides of the cervical vertebrae at the base of the skull on the muscles that go from the occipital ridge down to the base of the neck as it enters the shoulders. Apply gradual pressure along the muscles. Give this treatment special attention and slow, gentle pressure.

Your partner should have her head in a comfortable position. Try having your partner rest her forehead on a pillow so that as you press down you won't press her nose into the table. Resting the head on either side may also be comfortable.

## The Head Stroke

This is a long stroke which begins at the top of the head, moves down the back of the head, across the occipital ridge, along the muscles of the neck, down the trapezius and under the shoulder blades. Stand to whichever side of your

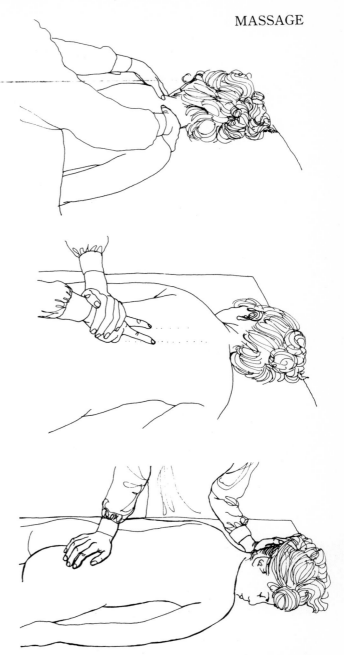

partner is most comfortable for you. Place your fingertips at the top of the head in the center. Apply some pressure by leaning your weight forward. Draw your fingertips down the back of the skull; then let your thumbs press into the occiput in the center groove, and slide them across the occiput and down the muscles at either side of the vertebrae of the neck. Slide your thumbs down the muscles, applying pressure as you do.

Slide your thumbs toward the outer crevice in the upper shoulders; then back toward each other and then to the spine. Now follow the inner edges of the shoulder blades, massaging the muscles between the shoulder blades and the spinal vertebrae. Then follow the half moon of the shoulder blades and bring your thumbs all the way down your partner's sides, to the table.

Use the first two fingers in your right hand to press on either side of the vertebrae at the base of the shoulder blades. Use the palm of your left hand to press on your right hand to help you exert more pressure with your fingertips. Pressing with your fingertips, slide your hands all the way up the vertebrae, from the shoulder blades to the top of the head and begin the head stroke again.

## The Spine Stretch

To do this, your friend's head should be facing away from you to the left. Standing to your partner's right side, take the heel of your right hand and lodge it under your friend's occipital ridge. Take the heel of your left hand and place it on the sacrum with your fingertips pointing toward the left hip. Gently and gradually apply pressure to the heels of both your hands, moving them very slightly outward so that you are stretching your friend's spine from top to bottom, by pressing the head up and the sacrum down. Release the pressure gradually.

## Back in the Foot

The next set of strokes relaxes the whole spine. Because there are nerve correspondence points for the back in the feet, massaging the feet is soothing to the spine. The arches of your feet correspond in the acupuncture system to your spine. Use your thumbs to make circles on the arches of your friend's feet by leaning way in and pressing. You can also use your thumbs and fingers to make a pleasant squeezing motion on the foot. Hold one foot in the palm of your hand and squeeze the arch with the fingers and thumb sliding the squeezing hand all the way from the person's heel down to their toes. Keep repeating the squeezing motion down the arch several times then do that stroking on the other foot. It's good to hold the foot slightly off the table so that their knee is bent a little. That way when you pull down on the foot you don't stretch the back of the knee uncomfortably.

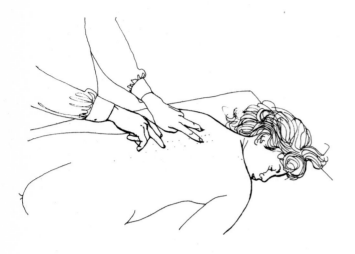

### The Waterfall

You begin at the top of the spine with the tips of the first two fingers of your right hand pressing into the muscles on either side of the vertebrae. You slide your fingertips about two or three inches down the muscles on either side of the spine. Then begin the same pressing, sliding motion with the first two fingertips of your left hand, covering again the area of your spinal muscles which your right hand has covered. Lift your right hand and slide the fingers of your left hand an inch or so farther down the back than your right hand. Now slide the fingertips of your right hand a few inches further down the back and keep repeating this alternating sliding and pressing with your fingertips on both sides of the spine. As one set of fingertips is pressing, raise the other off the back. Then start the motion with your other hand. On the receiving end the stroke correctly done will feel like a waterfall or having something smooth roll down your back.

### The Thumb Squeeze

Press the thumbs on each side of the spine between every vertebra from the neck down to the tailbone, and end with the sit bone caves. Press your thumbs toward each other in between each vertebra. Start at the base of the neck at the top of the shoulders, and work slowly down the back, taking care that you don't skip a vertebra.

### Crosshatching

The next stroke is called crosshatching. To do it, have your fingertips facing each other on top of your friend's spine. You can do this standing to one side of her waist or standing above her head. Lean your body weight into your fingertips slightly and with your fingertips spread wide apart and facing each other on the muscles on either side of the spine, press into the muscles. Now slide your fingertips toward each other and cross over the spine so that your hands meet and your fingertips mesh across the spine. Then separate your hands and drag them back out across the spine to the muscles again. Do this crossing motion up and down the whole spine with your fingertips.

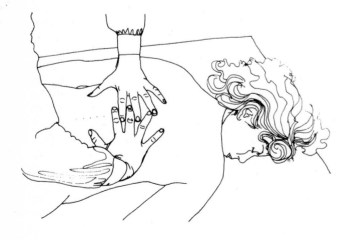

### The Spine Snake

Begin this movement at the tip of the coccyx by squeezing and lifting the skin at the base of the spine with your thumb and forefingers. Begin a rolling motion that you will continue from the base of your friend's spine all the way up her neck to the occipital ridge. By this point in the massage, some of the oil on the back has been absorbed. That's good because the spine snake is easier to do when the back's not too slippery. Gently grasp a roll of skin and then peel it or roll it along all the way up. On the receiving end, this is very releasing because it feels as though you are lifting nerves which may feel tense all the way up the back and relieving pressure from the spine.

### The Grand Finale

Back to basics. Simply repeat the basic back stroke to give a kind of continuity and security to the massage by covering the whole back again. Now you should both feel very relaxed and inspired to create full body strokes.

### Room for Creativity

You can invent full back strokes that connect different parts of the body to the back. For instance, by making circles with the palms of your hands, massage the arches of the feet and the base of the neck simultaneously; or massage the shoulder blades and the sacrum at the same time with a circular motion. Or massage the palms of your friend's hands and the base of her neck, or the palm of one hand and the sacrum, simultaneously. It's a pleasant sensation to have normally unconnected parts of your body connected by touch.

### Head to Toe

Stand at your partner's hips. Place your palms at the top of your partner's back on the shoulders. Lean your weight into your palms and draw your hands down the back to the hips, across the buttocks, and then down the back of each leg to the toes. Lift your hands when you have reached the toes. Return your palms to the upper back and repeat this downward stroke, covering the full length of your partner's body. You can also start this stroke at the top of the head.

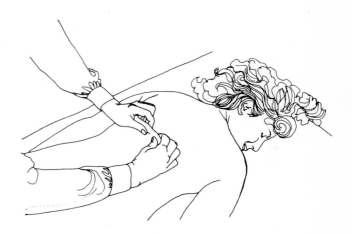

### Centering Energy

Stand to the left of your partner at approximately the middle of your partner's back. Place the palm of your right hand on your partner's sacrum and the palm of your left hand at the base of the neck where the neck moves into the shoulders. Applying no pressure, simply rest your palms there. Bend your knees slightly; center your energy; relax your breathing. Imagine that you are helping move the source of energy in your partner's body from the base of the spine, up the back and then out to the whole body, in the path of the kundalini energy. This cycle is rejuvenating and balancing.

Move your hands slowly away from your partner's back. Allow the person to lie still and relax awhile before getting up. Cover your friend with another beach towel or sheet to keep them warm while they relax in the glow of a well done massage.

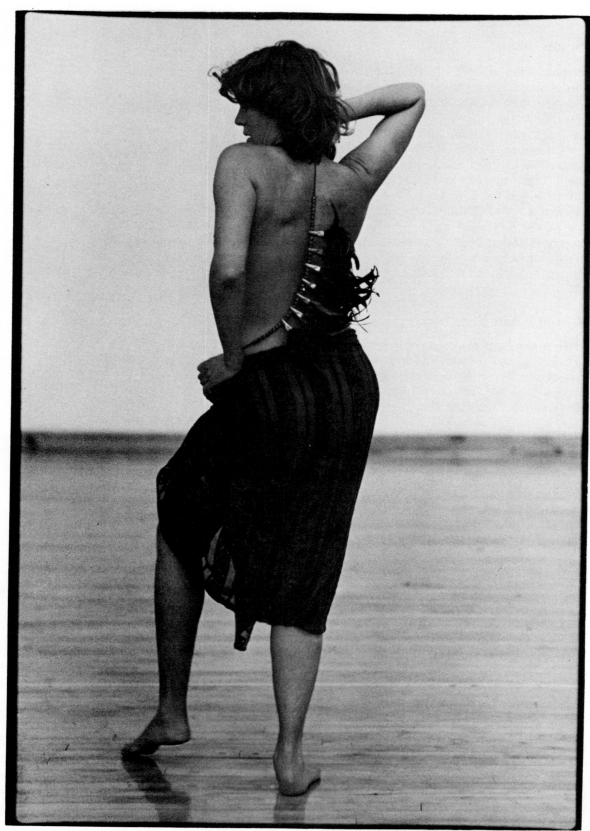

Diane Coleman

# A Dancer on Sensuality: Jamie Miller

Jamie Miller graduated from San Francisco State University with a Bachelor's Degree in Physical Education. She is now a performer, teacher and director. Her teaching includes yoga, creative movement, modern dance, acting, belly dancing and body alignment. She has performed with the San Francisco Mime Troupe, Bread and Roses, in dance programs for children, on television, at concerts, in nightclubs and in her own productions throughout the U.S. Miller lives in Oakland and teaches classes through Berkeley Moving Arts. In the following interview she talks about experience of sensuality, through the back and the whole body.

I have recently created a dance called The Erotic Suite. In some special sections of the dance I communicate entirely through my back. People are used to communicating with each other face to face. So often, when you communicate through your back, it's more erotic because it's more primal.

The long S-shape of the back is so beautiful. A straight back, which many people seem to think is the correct idea, is not particularly beautiful or comfortable. And it's not really possible to have a straight back. It's an injurious concept because the spine has a natural S-shape. The way to improve your spine is to visualize that S-shape always lengthening and releasing, rather than to think of it straightening. Thinking of a straight back tends to make you lock your pelvis. It's more pleasurable to think of the spine as long, growing and dynamic.

People's bodies change a great deal during belly dance training. The change is caused by two parts of the process. The first step is begun with exercises which encourage people to begin to feel and accept their bodies in a wholly pleasurable new way. In this beginning work, the focus is deeply personal and emphasizes each person's relationship to her or his own physical well being. The next step is more complex because it involves a growing self-awareness and ability to relate to others through performing.

Through performing, people gradually accept more responsiblity for their personal power by embracing and manifesting it. Performing is a pivotal step, and some people choose never to take it. But the people who decide to perform go through enormous personal growth because of it.

When I started performing it was in very sexist situations—in night clubs. Still for my own development, it felt healthy to proclaim my sexuality publicly. But the process was filled with a lot of anger and pain. Now there are enough people in the Bay Area who have become balanced in their attitudes about sexuality that it is possible to do a lot of belly dance performance without having to do it in sexist situations. New dancers are able to proclaim their sexuality publicly in healthier ways than were available to me when I began. But it was still a healthy thing for me to do even then, because it was embracing a part of myself that I thought I couldn't embrace in any other way. Even when the situation is distorted, as it is in night clubs, the movements themselves are so direct that they can't be untruthful. You can't distort belly dance movement that much. The movements of the spine, the pelvis, the legs and feet are basic and healthy. In belly dance you are trained to make a pure, rhythmic response to the music with your body. It is a very honest form.

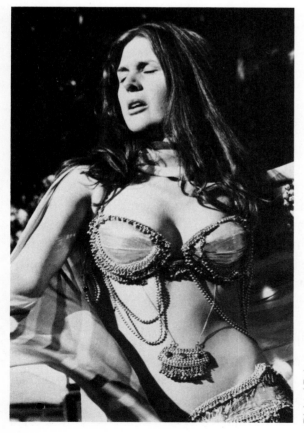

Richard Roberts

Although it may sound frightening there is also an enormous amount of power in overcoming the taboos and fears women accumulate to protect themselves from our culture's misogyny. Often when I dance I feel like a lion or a jaguar. There is so much animal strength to be found in expressing your sexuality full out. A lot of physical tensions that you feel or have felt at other times in your life are released through this process. You have more freedom. When you go outside the accepted norm, you find that there's a certain way in which you can't be hurt any more, because you've already taken the step. I associate this power with Kali, the Hindu goddess of time and death, and the kind of open expression of sexuality she symbolizes.

The Erotic Suite is an autobiographical story of my struggle to exist in this culture, and very much expresses my struggles as a woman and a dancer. I began it as part of a process which led to the creation of two works, The Erotic Suite and The Goddess Suite. I'm still in the process of creating The Goddess Suite and am just beginning to understand its structure, so it's hard for me to talk about it. I can talk about The Erotic Suite more easily. It is a series of dances based on the form of a belly dance. Together the dances tell a story. I had been directing a group of women and men; we worked together naked every week for six months. Two of us wanted to give a birthday present to another member of the group so we created dances. My dance was called The Fruit Song and became a piece in The Erotic Suite. That was in January. In May I performed The Erotic Suite for the first time, after it had been gestating for years.

There are ten parts to the suite: About You, Some Day, Satin Doll, For All We Know, Blanche's Dance, The Fruit Song, Love Tastes Like Strawberries, Minnie's Lament, Inside My Love, and Simple Things. The dance is set to Amercian popular music. I sing and do a strip to Satin Doll. And I sing a song called Love Tastes Like Strawberries, a West Indian ballad recorded by Miriam Makeba. Much of what the piece is about is the meaning of trying to claim our sexuality in this culture. The images are of the struggles I had to go through in that process. In one sense, it is my story as a woman. And it's also the story of a human being trying to be free. I'm happy to say that men love the dance as much as women do. That means a lot to me, because my aim as an artist and a human is to speak to other human beings, no matter what their age, or race, or sex.

Performing the suite marked a big change for me. It was the first time that I began to control what I want to say as an artist. After belly dancing in night clubs for quite a while, I started to teach. As a teacher I could create my own environment. I started producing Middle Eastern concerts of my own, hiring musicians, other professional belly dancers, and then my advanced students. Creating and performing The Erotic Suite enriched belly dancing for me in a way that I am sure wouldn't have happened otherwise. I've had years of training with many different kinds of dance and movement. I love belly dance, but it is limited. For instance, in belly dancing you don't use your legs very much. The legs are undercover. All the emphasis is on movements of the torso, the head, the arms and hands. I love to use my feet and legs in all kinds of ways. I am a Westerner: I'm used to big kicks, and I'm used to moving across large expanses of space. Being able to do this in The Erotic Suite means that when I belly dance, I don't feel limited by it.

It's interesting to see how my students respond to the movement training. I have a student who does a lot of African dance. She moves her spine and pelvis beautifully, but as soon as she puts on a belly dancing costume, she freezes, because she thinks of belly dancing as specifically sexual. I suspect she feels that belly dancing is exhibitionist, whereas African dance probably feels more communal, more tribal to her.

One of the original aims of belly dancing was to exhibit yourself. It's a positive urge to express self-love under comfortable circumstances. Being forced to exhibit yourself in unpleasant surroundings is another matter. Belly dancing as we know it is an expression of a culture in which women's existence depended completely on man. A woman in the ancient Middle East could only be a wife or a whore. The women who danced in the cities were whores. If you were in a harem, you were supported at the Sultan's whim. Belly dance still has reference to that slavery. You can do the same dance for all kinds of different reasons. Women danced for each other in the harem while a woman was giving birth. Then the belly dancing could feel very free and positive. If they were forced to dance for the Sultan, or for other reasons, then they weren't free. It isn't the form or the movement that is bad or good, it's the intention behind the movement, and the situation of the dancing.

The fact that belly dancing has flourished in so many cultures is an affirmation of its roots as a pure celebration of the life force, the movement of the womb, and the female principle. The form itself is probably older than any patriarchy. Many of us assume that feeling good about ourselves is bad for the tribe, that it's selfish or against the communal spirit. Consequently, people can take dance classes for years yet never own the movement. They can move exquisitely during a class, but think of that movement as a form into which they must fit themselves. That's often a serious shortcoming of Western dance training, which occurs because ours is a secular culture. If you look to the dance forms of the East, or of Africa, you see expressions of cultures where fragmentation of sensuality and spirituality has not taken place as it has here. There it is understood that when you embrace your own beauty, you're expressing the beauty of the universe. In this culture we seem to feel that there's a conflict between the good of the group and the good of the individual. Dance, for me, is a spiritual experience. I feel that when I embrace my self, which includes my sexuality, fully, then I embrace my sacredness. In its highest form, that's what belly dancing enables. In its highest form that's what any form of dance does. It's up to each person to choose the particular form they want to use to manifest that energy.

My Fruit Song dance begins with me wearing a wine-red velvet and chiffon veil flung over my hips like a sarong. I wear a green feather necklace and I'm bare breasted. I pick up a bowl laden with fruit and do the "camel walk" around the stage area, then down the center of the stage. Then I kneel before the audience and offer them the fruit. The camel walk is exquisite, because it is a deeply integrated movement—an undulation of the spine which runs through the pelvis down into the legs and feet—through the whole body. When I do it I feel like the pictures I've seen of women in the Caribbean, or in Africa with heavy packages on their heads.

I think that if I could go around the world and get people really relaxed and turn on belly dance music, most people would respond naturally by belly dancing. These movements are natural to all of us. When people get relaxed, feeling good about themselves, accepting their body moving sensually and erotically, they're going to end up belly dancing. Belly dancing is like making love. When people have trouble making love, most of the time it's because they're nervous about themselves. It's not that the knowledge isn't in them, it's that they're mentally upset because they don't measure up to some pre-

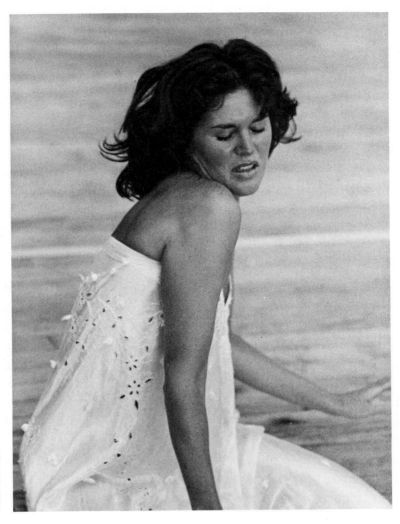

Diane Coleman

conceived image of what they should be.

When I perform, I feel as though the audience is my lover. My task is to surrender myself to my lover. That's why I love to do it so much. The audience is like a big gourmet feast and the performer just gets to eat! The real challenge of the performance is to have the courage to eat all you want, but not to get off center and overindulge. In other words, to use the audience without letting it sweep you away. There's a delicate balance. The task of the dancer is to open her or himself so that the energy of the universe can flow through. In this way the performer and the audience embrace and become one.

One of the things that the back can communicate is fear of other people, or a desire to be separate from other people: turning your back on someone. After I dance The Fruit Song, I come up stage toward the audience. Then I turn my back on them, and go into an attitude of mourning. It's like one phase of making love. When you make love, you accept death as well as life, and for me the transition between my Fruit Song dance and Minnie's Lament is about the pain of that acceptance. After you open up as much as you do when you make love, there comes the pain of contracting. That's just part of being alive. I think Minnie's Lament is about that pain which I express through my back a lot.

It's still another kind of beauty, maybe a beauty that's harder for us to accept. But it's part of being alive. I now have the idea that I'm always supposed to be open to people, so when I contract it's become hard for me to accept myself. But I'm learning that turning my back can be a constructive way of protecting myself.

The pelvis is a bridge between the spine and the legs. If the pelvis is blocked, then energy can't flow through the whole body. That blockage is the cause of a great deal of lower back tension and pain. Many people have knee problems. These are often linked with the movement of the lower back, with the pelvis as the bridge between the two. The knee problems get better if you release and lengthen your spine. People should check to see whether they stand with locked knees. As soon as you release the knees, you release your pelvis. The upper spine is related to the heart chakra and so is central to our emotions and to our capacity for love.

I've worked with a lot of strippers and I think that their impulse with stripping is an honestly pure celebration of the body. I'm thinking of older women I've worked with who didn't have any other avenue in our culture for that kind of expression. I once taught a class on dressing and undressing for men and women where we explored what that meant to us. It was very exciting! It was a chance to feel the real impulse for stripping: revealing yourself to other people. I think the reason that a lot of men in an audience get angry when women strip is that they would like to get up there and strip too. Men often get angry that women have those kinds of opportunities, limited as they might be, to express their sexuality.

It's always wonderful to see people who genuinely and honestly enjoy their bodies. Most men who are able to enjoy their bodies in this culture do it only through competitive sports. Competition is part of women's self-expression too, because we're supposed to look good to catch a man. But women are much more fortunate in being allowed to enjoy the texture of our clothes, colors, make-up, and more daily sensuality, frivolity and play.

This makes me think of another student who, when we worked on deep pelvic movement, told me how inhibited she felt. She said she felt as though someone was present judging her. I told her to tell that person to get out of her pelvis! The kind of association she made happens a lot when people work deeply within themselves. They find they do not own aspects of themselves. It's a powerful step to free your body. In teaching, the greatest thing I do is to give my students complete permission to embrace themselves. That seems to be the hardest thing for people, including me, to do. And yet that embrace is the struggle, the door to joy.

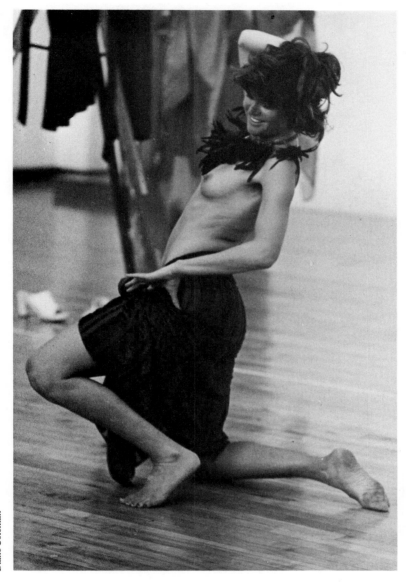

Diane Coleman

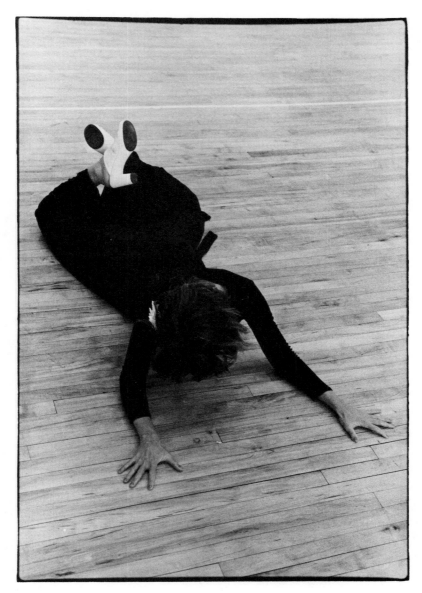

Diane Coleman

# A Survey

In the process of gathering information on attitudes about the back, I decided to take an informal poll to discover how people felt about the back's sensuality. Stephanie Mills and I spent a few days phoning friends, and saying: "I am taking a survey. Do you think the back is sensual?" The people we called were told that their answers might be used in the book and that they could, if they chose, remain anonymous. We learned that you don't have to be a belly dancer to enjoy your back, and that attitudes about the back are as individual as any other opinions. These are the responses of the people who were brave enough to share their philosophy with us.

Eleanor Smith, editor and writer
**Sensual, yes, probably erotic, no.**

Ron Rudolph, no title necessary
**Backs are essentially sensual, or sensually essential; either one, they're great.**

Jim Harding, energy expert
**Hmm. Not at rest.**

Karen Cooper, Director of Film Forum, New York
**Sure.**

Anonymous
**When you can't get the front.**

Enid Goldman, journalist
**I think the lower back is.**

Kathy Bartoloni, international liaison
**Only without clothes . . . it's especially sensual if it's female, if it's got your stereotypic, spaghetti-strap, lowcut dress. I don't think that backs that show tan marks of any sort are sensual. I'll even take a little hair on the back of the man who bit me.**

Betty Lynn Moulton, psychologist
**Yes, I believe I do, depending on whose back. Also it feels good.**

Jeff Jones, musician
**The back of what? Yeah, I've never really thought too much about it. But both from a passive as well as an active viewpoint, it's definitely sensual. At least mine is. I would rate it next to feet, very high on a sensuality scale.**

John Diamante, gardener
**Yes. Even noble in some cases, often erotic, and as I say, basic to the working class.**

Jeanne Campbell, stockbroker
**Absolutely. Any part of your body that's ignored is heavily sensual: If someone pays attention to your underside, you think they love you.**

Robin Flower, musician
**Every part of the body is sensual.**

Mary Wings, comic book author and ceramicist
**Absolutely. I love my spaniel's back the best.**

John Neumann, metal craftsman and musician
**I love backs because they are smooth and good to bite. Some backs, that is, yours, for example . . .**

Dr. Pat Grosh, computer scientist, psychologist and greyhound breeder
**It's got to be. It's a lot closer to your erogenous zones than your head is. Besides, few rubs feel better than a back rub.**

David Chadwick, Zen priest
**It depends on the person. But to me, anything is sensual. Whatever turns anybody on is great.**

Peter Berg, editor
**The human back . . . no question about it.**

Judith Hill, astrologer
**Shoulders are! And backs of necks. I am a secret vampire, I think. And did you know Leos are supposed to have the most beautiful backs?**

Hallie Iglehart, witch
**Yes! The back is one of the most sensual parts of the body. I discovered this when I was twelve years old in summer camp. Two other girls and I took turns giving one another back rubs with Jergens lotion. I often wondered why we couldn't stop rubbing one another's back—now I know!**

Jamie Nelson, managing editor
**Is the back sensual? Oh, definitely. Unquestionably. I think the back in motion is wonderful to watch, nicer to hold, and best to exercise.**

Sarah Wingfield, publicist

**The back? Of course backs are sensual. They're all full of contours, and they're strong, and when you curl up in bed next to a back, you can nestle like spoons. Also you can dig your fingers into them.**

Merlin Stone, writer

**Apart from the rest of the body? If I were presented with a back by itself, no. But any part of the body can be sensual. If a person turns me on I could touch anywhere and it would be sensual.**

Mary Pougiales, deputy D.A.

**Yes. It's like stories about crocodiles and alligators; when you scratch their stomachs, they go to sleep. Well, it's that kind of feeling.**

Paul Chignell, police officer

**I would echo her statements.**

Walter Carey, hairdresser

**The back is probably one of the most sensually relaxing areas of the body—when touched properly. I mean, anything is sensual if it's touched sensually—a lost art these days. I'm in a position to know about sensuality because in my profession I touch people all day long. If my touch were wrong, I'd be out of business by now!**

Charlene Spretnak, author

**I like backs.**

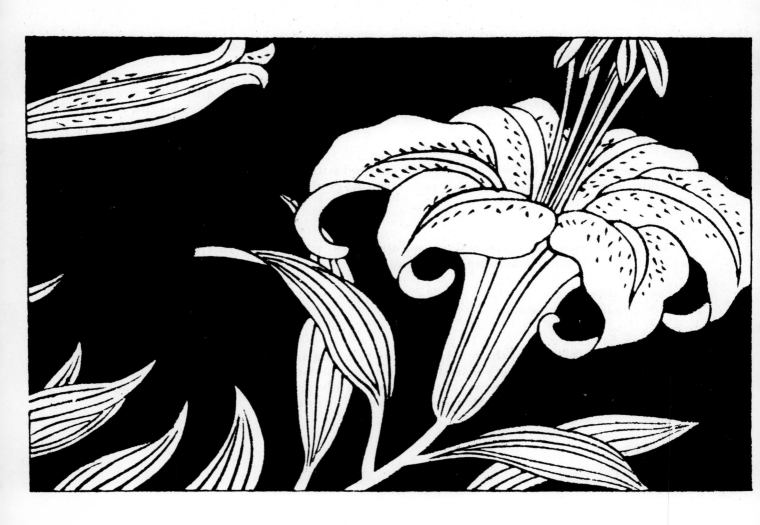

# Sex & Backaches

The back is clearly key to a great deal of sensual pleasure. Lower back strength, flexibility and pelvic agility are basic ingredients of movement during most sexual intimacy. Just as low back constriction during sex can cause back pain, comfortable pelvic movement during sex can also be preventive back pain exercise. For people with low back pain, therefore, the sex act is superb exercise, and the more prolonged it is, the better.

If you have a healthy spine, from time to time be aware of your movements and your body alignment during sex. Tension during sex or any activity, is neutral: your muscles may either be tense as a result of excitement and pleasure, or as a result of anxiety and distress. The second form of tension is, of course, the one to avoid, not only to insure your emotional balance but also to preserve your physical health. If you feel any pain or discomfort in your body, especially in your back during sex be sure to shift your position and/or that of your partner so that you can move more easily. If you have chronic back ache or temporary pain from injury, the positions described in this chapter should enable you to enjoy sex anyway.

Back pain, especially low back pain, is often connected with psychological ambivalence about sex. Examine your feelings about your own sexuality and that of your partner to uncover any emotional sexual stress. Left unexplored, these tensions can prevent your sexual satisfaction. If explored gently and wisely, either alone, or with a friend or therapist, they can usually be eliminated. A happier sex life is the reward. Remember also that if your ambivalence is about your sexuality with a partner, you are not in that pickle alone. It is the relationship which should be undergoing therapy. Neither one of you can solve the problems single-mindedly. Respectful mutual examination of the relationship, or couple therapy, usually helps.

You may, however, not be in psychological turmoil. You may simply have been in an accident and, therefore, need to be physically careful of your back during sex. Pay close heed to the suggestions which follow and you should have a happy recovery period.

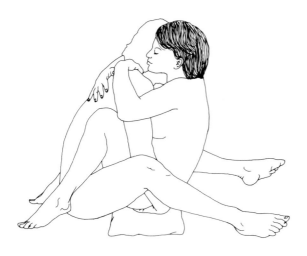

## POSITIONS AFTER INJURY

Immediately after an injury, of course, it is best to refrain from sex temporarily. When you are feeling good enough to experiment try some of the following positions. Ideally a person with a back ache should keep a mild "S" curve in the spine. There are many ways a partner can adjust to this position. An interlocking "S" position is best if both partners have back aches.

### Sit Ups

A position which provides back protection for both people can be achieved sitting up. Have your hips and knees flexed. One person sits inside the embrace of the other. The woman should sit on a pillow in order to be slightly higher than her partner; this will circumvent strain on the partner's spine.

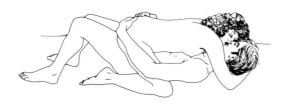

### Staying On Top Of It

If only one of you has a back ache, the ache-less partner can lie flat on his back while the other straddles in a position to maintain a spinal "S" curve. If you're on top, you can lessen the burden of your weight by placing your elbows beside your partner's shoulders. Be sure to keep your torso inclined forward to lessen the curve in your lower back.

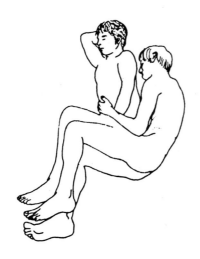

### Spoons

This position always reminds me of spoons in a drawer, very cozy. It is also like sitting in someone's lap while lying on your side. You can flex your hips, knees and spine easily in this protected position and minimize pressure on the back.

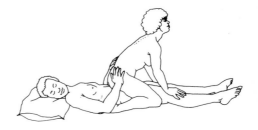

## Half Sit Up

If the woman only has a back ache her partner can lie on his back. She straddles his pelvis facing his feet. Easing her body weight by leaning on her pelvis, she leans her torso forward and uses her leg muscles for pelvic movement.

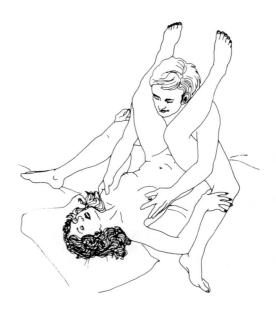

## Leg Rest

One partner lies on her back with her legs on the partner's shoulders. The partner's arms can be under the legs as in the illustration. Or you can support your partner's legs under your arms against your sides if the first position is too strenuous.

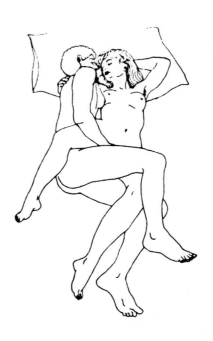

## Profiles

This position is usually comfortable for both people. Lie on your back, knees bent. Your partner lies on her side with hips and knees flexed in a sitting position. If you are lying on your back intertwine all your legs so that your upper leg is draped around your partner's waist and your lower leg is in between your partner's thighs.

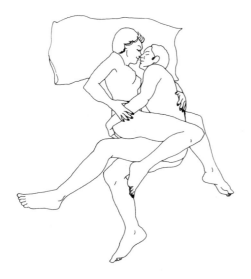

## Face to Face

Both people lie on their sides facing each other. She wraps her legs around the hips of her partner as though she were sitting on his lap. He flexes his hips and knees so that his thighs brace under her buttocks. Both people should be able to move easily and avoid lower back strain in this position.

After back injury or strain, downward pressure on your spine is usually quite uncomfortable. So if you have a sore back, any position in which you are on top and, therefore, free to adjust your spine easily and free of the pressure of your partner's body weight, is desirable.

## Strengthening the Pelvic Floor

Strong, supple pelvic floor muscles are extremely important for a woman's sexual agility and comfort. To strengthen your pelvic floor, do simple vaginal muscle contractions several times during the day. Gradually work up to about fifty or a hundred contractions per day. To see if you are contracting the right muscles, test by stopping and releasing the flow during urination several times. You will learn to feel these muscles distinctly. For both men and women, masturbating can be excellent for developing your pelvic floor muscles. Be sure you don't constrict your breathing as you do.

## Neck Pain During Sex

Whether your whole back hurts or just your neck you will want to follow the same position precautions. For neck pain, however, you must be especially careful to avoid extending the cervical spine. This is difficult because it goes against your natural impulse to arch your head and neck back during very pleasurable moments. But to avoid straining your neck, keep your chin tucked under, as close to your chest as is comfortable.

**The world's greatest contraceptive is the back ache.**
—Twentieth century folklore

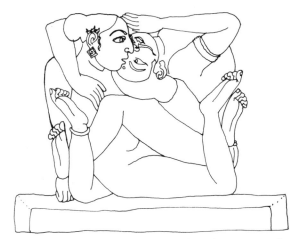

An eighteenth century Nepalese sexual posture called Cakra Asana, said to affect the spinal energies in a powerful way. Not recommended for those with back problems.

## Massage, Saunas, Jacuzzi

For any low back strain, or just to relax before sex, massages, saunas, and Jacuzzi baths are excellent treats. You soothe away the tensions of the day which can distract you from sensuality, and you relax tense muscles so you can move freely.

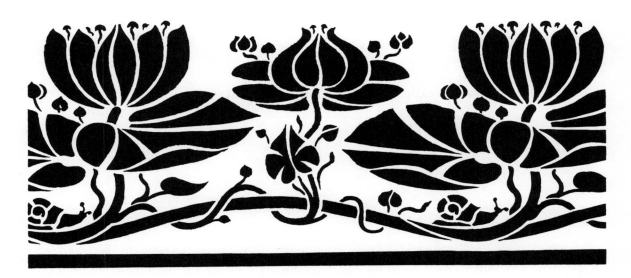

We differ from ordinary machines, however, in one marvelous respect—we are self-repairing.[19]

—Maggie Lettvin, MAGGIE'S BACK BOOK


The body has an endless longing to improve and to work.

—Marion Rosen

# V
# Self-Healing after Injury

# AFTER INJURY — SECTION V: CONTENTS

**Whose Responsibility is Health?**

**Emergency Guidelines**

**Relieving Pain After Injury:** Meg Stern

**An Orthopedic Surgeon:** Richard H. Cobden, M.D.

**An Acupuncturist:** Dr. Evon Karanoff

**A Chiropractor:** Dr. Alice Francis

**Exercises After Injury:** Phase One of Healing: Isometrics; The Pelvic Tilt; Knee Lift; Torso Stretch; Sacrum Roll; Partial Sit Up; Torso Hang; Phase Two of Healing: Knee Kiss; Leg Scissors; Walking Backward; Neck Lift; Blade Squeeze; Arm Stretch; Standing Squat; Cervical Stretches; Small Cobra; Wing Back Stretch; The Shrug; Corrective Rests; Wall Press; Kneeling Ballet; Relaxation; Phase Three of Healing: More Rigorous Exercise; Three Phases of the Cow-Cat; Jump Rope; Swimming; Variety Is

The regimen I adopt shall be for the benefit of my patients according to my ability and judgment, and not for their hurt or for any wrong. I will give no deadly drug to any, though it be asked of me . . . Whatsoever house I enter, there will I go for the benefit of the sick, refraining from all wrongdoing or corruption, and especially from any act of seduction, of male or female, of bond or free.

—from the Hippocratic Oath

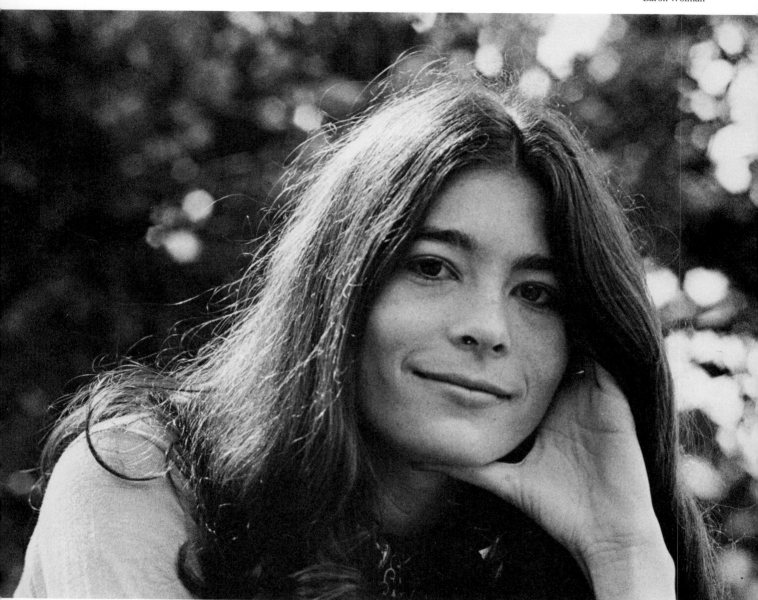

Stephanie Mills

# Whose Responsibility is Health?
## Stephanie Mills

In this section several approaches to healing an injury are presented. You may want to choose one or combine several for the best treatment.

In the Resources section, attorney Richard Sindell deals with some of your options for compensation if your health practitioner fails you and is at fault. Sindell gives an excellent picture of what's involved in a legal attempt to win financial compensation for personal injury resulting from someone else's negligence, whether the negligent party is one's physician or dentist, another driver, or the manufacturer of an unsafe product. He also describes the Worker's Compensation system, which attempts to recompense people who are injured on the job.

As you may infer from the chapter, a personal injury lawsuit will land you squarely in the hands of the legal and medical professions, and will require you to seek your relief according to their rules. In our opinion, such lawsuits are usually a last resort. Certainly there are cases where wrong has been done and justice should be sought. And the money you may be awarded might ameliorate your life after an injury, but it cannot restore all your injury has cost you. Furthermore, suing in cases of medical malpractice, however justified, deepens the rift between physicians and patients, and drives up the costs of medical services. This is not a happy situation.

To us, it makes better sense to try to avoid those situations altogether by taking responsibility for your own health to the greatest extent possible. This means, in part, using the services of medical and holistic practitioners as an active, informed, and cooperative client. And doing this implies rethinking traditional roles.

As attorney, Jerry Green, has pointed out in several articles, many of us have come to regard health as a product delivered by certified physicians, and are consequently disappointed when it's not forthcoming. Doctor Jeff Kane writes that the rate of damage has not risen as high as the rate of disappointment, and this is where the suits begin. Sindell points out that neither hospitals nor doctors guarantee that you will recover. This isn't always stated, and it is hard to accept. Doctors' and hospitals' responsibility is to deliver competent services; that competence is defined by locally accepted standards of medical practice. Nobody can guarantee recovery because healing, as Dr. Segal says, is something of a mystery. Your physician may bind up your wounds, but it is, finally, the life force that animates the healing process.

Coming to terms with this mystery, and being willing to pursue our health without benefit of guarantees runs counter to popular mythology. Not so long ago, M.D.'s, in attempt to protect our modesty, would say, "Your body is just a machine to me", and would order us off their turf by telling us that "a little bit of knowledge is a dangerous thing," not conceding that no knowledge is even more dangerous and that their knowledge, too, has its limits.

This attitude encouraged a certain passivity about personal health. If we were ignorant machines, and the doctor an omniscient mechanic, the annual physical was our tune up. We even could count on replacement parts. We expected professional solutions to our mechanical problems. Even problems resulting from the way we ran the machine could be solved by hiring a good mechanic. The only place the analogy failed was that no complaints to the dealer, or trade-ins were possible. Given this model, we were bound to be disappointed; we aren't machines, but beings with mind and spirit.

After enough of us woke up with sponges in our stomachs, or got sicker as a result of unexpected miracle drug synergies, or discovered we were DES daughters, or saw friends and relatives wasted by medical mistakes, many of us came to mistrust our physicians.

Still, it is hard to abandon our technological optimism; and compared to our traditional medicine, holistic approaches may seem somehow unorthodox. The irreducible fact of the matter is that either approach to health contains some risks. Unavoidable risks of life itself include pain and death. We just keep trying to get around them in spite of the fact that sooner or later, ten out of ten of us will die anyway. Ivan Illich, in MEDICAL NEMESIS: *The Expropriation of Health*, gives the bottom line: if we are to regain control of our own lives, we must be ready to risk some pain. Jeff Kane says that, "Personal power is not bought, sold, given, or taken: it is assumed."

One might also say that to regain personal power over our health, we must also risk joy—the joy of living life as fully integrated beings, not as clever machines in need of constant maintenance by someone else. This means that the primary responsibility for your health is yours. Assuming this power doesn't leave much room for negligence. It means entering into a learning relationship with your practitioner, and making agreements about your respective responsibilities in that relationship as it develops; it means a knowledgeable acceptance of risks.

This agreement, or plan, can take the form of a contract with the practitioner. It is a way for each of you to clarify your expectations, your limitations, and your mutual responsibilities at the outset. You may each want to revise the agreement as your relationship progresses. Developing such an agreement with a physician or holistic practitioner is a way to evaluate the practitioner and to avoid many disappointments, and it suggests a means of recourse if the contract isn't honored. Such agreements are particularly relevant to holistic practices, although forming them with M.D.'s would probably be conducive to better healing and feeling.

It is important to understand that holistic healing is not the practice of medicine. Generally speaking, holistic practice deals with the health of a particular individual, and facilitates that individual's interaction with his or her environment. Medical practice deals with disease and common symptoms. It is the diagnosis and treatment of recognized disease entities. Medicine is logical, holistic practice empirical; the dichotomy between the two philosophies is twenty centuries old. Both approaches are useful; it's not an either/or question. If you suffer a major wound, you probably should head for the nearest emergency ward, rather than to your polarity therapist. If you have more time and are interested in learning how to achieve balance for optimum functioning and avoidance of disease, you probably want a holistic practitioner.

You have options in your responsibility for your health. To exercise them, you may want to choose a physician carefully. To find a physician, ask your friends. Their recommendations can help you avoid shopping your way through the medical society's roster. Ideally, your physician should be a special kind of friend, a friend you want to know all your life. He or she should be willing to answer your questions, to supply an accurate diagnosis of your condition, to tell you the meaning of the results of any tests performed, to tell you the pros and cons of the treatment he or she recommends, and alternatives to it, along with the reasons for his or her preferences. Your doctor should be willing to give you complete information about any drugs prescribed, and be willing to stop any examination or procedure at any time, if you request. Your doctor should be willing to wait for a second medical opinion before performing any elective surgery. Your doctor should treat you with respect.

Above all, you should feel that you can trust your doctor. This trust is crucial to healing, and the adversary relationship, which is deepened by malpractice suits, works against this trust. Some doctors have opted out of the adversary business and "go bare"— they practice without malpractice insurance, and try to establish a trusting and cooperative relationship with their patients. These M.D.'s are candid; they admit their limitations and their fallibility, and they tell their patients that they carry no insurance. This honest acknowledgement of risk helps prevent the disappointments which lead to suits. And this pioneering approach seems to be working well.

Making contracts with holistic practitioners or developing a mature relationship with your physician assumes the ability to make informed choices. Given our general level of confusion about health, that ability is rare. The medical mystique, the indemnified life, and sue-me, sue-you approach to problem solving continues to dominate our thinking.

But in the long run, we think that the solution to a lot of health problems will be found not in hospitals, or in court, but at the individual and social levels. We can affect our individual lives immediately; we just have to do what we can to take care of ourselves. Some insurance companies are even rewarding people for taking a preventive approach to their health by offering policy discounts to people who exercise regularly. But our socially determined environment, with its noise, stress, artificiality, and pervasive bio-hazards is an enormous factor to contend with. All the alfalfa sprouts and yoga in the world may fail to keep you healthy if you work in a chemical plant, or live downwind from one.

The attempt to lead a healthier life is part of a shift in values away from planetary pathology, a small beginning step. Developing environmental and political consciousness, and beginning to work on some of these issues is a bigger step, but quite as necessary. The ultimate goal is to live as wholly on the earth as we can; maintaining and enjoying our fullest humanity, in mind, body and spirit is a good place to start.

**Sources:**

Jerry Green, "Contracts With Your Doctor?" *New Realities*, Vol. II, No. I. And "Liability and Holistic Health Practice," *Yoga Journal*, September 1978.
Jeff Kane, M.D., "Insurance and the Abandonment of Responsibility," *CoEvolution Quarterly*, Spring 1979.
Boston Women's Healthbook Collective, OUR BODIES, OUR SELVES; Simon & Schuster.
Ivan Illich, MEDICAL NEMESIS: *The Expropriation of Health*; Bantam.

# Emergency Guidelines

In this section I describe some of the basic guidelines to emergency treatment of back problems. It is beyond the limits of this book to provide a manual on emergency procedures, and you'll need to study a good text or take a course on the subject to become really qualified to administer treatment. In general, however, the following guidelines will help you approach problem situations and give you a better understanding of the dynamics of emergency back care.

## Pain

Pain is our bodies' most urgent warning signal. Acute pain is a message that we must change our condition or environment quickly. Chronic pain is a message that we need to alter something in our way of life. Dealing with pain is often like solving a many layered mystery. The causes are not always obvious and many attempts may be made to find them before the actual root of the pain is discovered. Sometimes the causes are obvious, and the only block to relieving our misery is reluctance to make the decision to eradicate the cause.

Pain causes the muscles to tighten in an effort to alleviate it. Often knots or muscle spasms result. The constriction of muscles causes pressure on blood vessels, which results in decreased blood flow to the tense area. This leads to a localized anemia called ischemia. Ischemic pain results from a lack of circulation of oxygen and nutrients to the tightened area. This causes more pain and tension, and a terrible cycle is set up. The goal of pain treatments is to short circuit this escalating cycle.

Dolorology is a new medical specialty devoted to the treatment of chronic pain. Dolorologists use a wide variety of techniques, from drugs and surgery to meditation and hypnosis. Many dolorologists are exploring a new theory of the transmission of pain called "gate control." This theory supposes a pain "gate" in the spinal cord; relief is based on somehow closing this gate to prevent pain signals from reaching the brain. Pain impulses move along two types of nerve fibers, A-delta and C fibers, to the two bundles of nerve fibers on either side of the spine, the spinothalamic tract. If the impulses travel up to the brain stem and the thalamus, they are perceived as pain. Techniques such as acupuncture, hypnosis and electrical stimulation to change the impulses along the spinal cord in brain stem to close the "gate" have significantly relieved chronic pain in many cases.

Another medical discovery related to pain control is the presence of natural opiates in the body called enkephalins. Electrical stimulation of the nerves can release enkephalins in the brain and therefore help to relieve pain. Through focused meditation or biofeedback we can also trigger production of enkephalins for healing any disorder. People with less enkephalin in their systems may have higher susceptibility to pain.

If you have acute pain as a result of an accident you can apply emergency techniques to relieve it temporarily. Descriptions of a few treatments are included, but you can also find thorough books on this topic. Two useful texts are: *Emergency Medical Guide*, John Henderson, M.D., McGraw-Hill, paperback; and *Emergency First Aid*, Charles Mosher, M.D., Consumer Guide.

## In Case of Accident

If a person is in an accident which has shifted or broken a vertebra, your immediate goal is to prevent damage to the spinal cord. Broken bones will heal with few if any ill effects in the long term. However, if the spinal cord is injured permanent damage almost always results. To avoid damage to the injured person's spinal cord do not move them unless absolutely necessary.

You may need to clear the person's breath passage. Bend the neck as little as possible; don't lift the neck or head. Keep the neck stationary while you lift the jaw and tongue to ease their breathing.

Even if there are no visible signs of back injury you should assume it and proceed accordingly to prevent possible damage to the spinal cord. If the person is conscious tell her or him to lie still. Do not move an unconscious victim unless her or his life is in danger from remaining where they lie. Try to be sure the spine and neck are in a straight line. If the victim must be moved, put her or him on a flat surface and wrap cloth strips around them to hold them securely in place on the flat surface. Do not put a pillow under the head. Keep the person flat and still. Keep the back and head from rolling to the side by cushioning them at the sides of the body or by holding the head motionless. If the victim is sitting, support the head to keep it from moving.

Have an ambulance called or get a medical specialist to treat the victim. Keep holding the head to prevent injury while splints or straps are being attached.

If the victim has a fractured neck he or she should be placed on the back on the stretcher. With a fractured back the victim is placed face down on a rigid stretcher.

## Less Catastrophic Problems

The best body position to relieve lower back strain is to lie flat on the back with the knees bent and lower legs supported by pillows. Heat on the back helps relax muscle spasm. The patient should rest and move as little as possible until the pain subsides. The back can be taped or braced by a professional to hold it in place. Steam baths and heat pads are also good for muscle strains.

Cold packs are usually more effective on pinched nerves than heat. Use ice bags or water treatments.

If you move incorrectly or are thrown off balance and you pull a back muscle, squatting immediately afterwards can head off severe injury. Relax your chin toward your chest; bend your knees with your feet flat on the floor; tilt your pelvis forward; curl your back forward and lower yourself into a squatting position. You can gently bounce up and down a few inches by pushing up and releasing your leg muscles. Bounce fifteen or twenty times and then stand up to rest. Repeat this cycle several times an hour. If squatting is uncomfortable, lie on your back and bring your knees over your chest. Move the knees gently into this position several times to relax and stretch your muscles. Gentle stretching loosens the muscle spasm and lessons pressure on the nerves. Gentle massage is also releasing to sprains and strains. These are techniques which also help relieve sciatica.

Maggie Lettvin, in the book THE BEAUTIFUL MACHINE (Ballantine), says her technique for instant relief of back muscle strain is to hang from a bar. Clamp an exercise bar in a doorway, high enough to chin yourself on. If your back "goes out" stand on a chair; hold onto the bar tightly; bend your knees slowly; and gradually lower yourself so your feet are not supporting your body weight. Hold this hanging position for about a half a minute, and stand up. Repeat this hanging release several times. Tilt and stretch one hip, then the other. If you do this soon enough after your strain you can be completely relieved.

Certain postures are helpful to relieve the pain of muscle strain or pinched nerves. When you sleep on your back, lie with a pillow under your hips to ease the arch in the lower back and with a pillow under your knees. Keep a pillow between your legs to support your knees if you prefer to lie on your side. When you are sitting, place your feet on a stool to keep the hips and knees flexed. If your back pain is localized on one side of your body, you may relieve it somewhat while standing by elevating the foot on the painful side, using a small stool. Remember that recovery has certain phases and you must respect them in order to heal well. The first stage calls for rest, until there is little or no pain. In the second stage, do mild exercises to begin restoring your muscles. The last stage is to do preventive exercises as part of your daily routine in order to avoid future problems.

## Headache Relief

Headaches are often a result of upper back and neck tension. Tension headaches are caused by prolonged contraction of the muscles of the head, neck and upper back. Heat and massage on the sore areas is helpful. Acupressure point therapy or shiatsu, is quite beneficial. Changing the elements of your life which produce the headaches though, is the most effective treatment.

The throbbing pain of migraine headaches is caused by dilation of the blood vessels around the brain. To relieve this pain somewhat lie flat on your back with a pillow under your head in a quiet, dark room. Move as little as possible to prevent dizziness. Apply an ice bag at the base of the skull and cold compresses to the forehead. Drinking strong hot tea with lots of honey can relieve weakness and nausea.

## Acupressure Points

There are many explanations for the remarkable, natural effectiveness of pressure point therapy. Some people say the points release pinched nerves. Some people claim the pressure blocks oxygen supply to the areas and thus prevents the nerves from continuing a spasm. Others theorize that the pain is caused by blocks in the flow of electromagnetic currents in our systems.

Some important body points to treat to relieve headaches are the occipital ridge at the base of the skull, the trapezius shoulder muscles, the temples, the muscles at the back of the neck and all the muscle areas on either side of the spine, including those of the sacrum.

## Social Pain

The major cause of chronic pain, especially head and back pain, is social stress and tension. Our bodies need to release tension as it develops. If we are prevented from this release we develop frozen muscles and our tissues, stiffened into defensive position, are always just on the verge of nervous discharge. The combination of the emotional depression which results from pain and the constant defensive attitude produced by holding our bodies on the edge of release accounts for the fact that pain gradually destroys the personality. You become irritable and less able to perceive the environment in a balanced way.

Because our modern society is constantly stressful, with loud noises, fast vehicles, hard pavements, speedy schedules and social restrictions on our emotions in daily life, we need urgently to counteract these stresses in order to maintain our health. We must find the time and the environments in which to express a wide range of pent-up emotion. Our bodies need a chance to live out the impulses we hold in abeyance during most social situations. Since we can't, realistically, hit someone who mistreats us at work, we may need to use punching bags or pillows to vent our natural reactions. Our bodies also have a natural impulse to run from threatening situations in which we are often expected to remain during a crisis. I imagine one of the reasons running is such a popular activity these days is that it allows us to express this daily restricted response.

Exercise and emotional expression are good preventive measures for problems caused by today's lifestyles. We also need to encourage our children to move well and often. Even young people's lifestyles are becoming more sedentary and physically restricted. If we encourage a wide range of healthy movement in our children we will help them circumvent adult health problems.

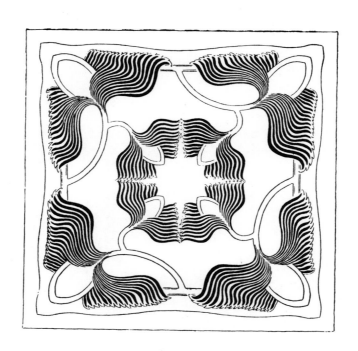

# Relieving Pain After Injury: Meg Stern

Meg Stern works with people who have back problems, teaching classes in the San Francisco Bay Area, and she has developed a special exercise program for people with back injuries. In this chapter she talks about her approach to pain relief and healing. She describes her work as "an alternative to traditional medical treatment of back problems—an alternative to living with pain."

In my classes I offer specific exercises and positions to relieve low back and neck pain. I never recommend an exercise that causes any pain. I show how to cope with everyday life in ways that help to relieve and reduce pain: how to stand, sit, walk, sleep, carry and lift; how to avoid the discomfort that sneezing, coughing, or laughing can produce after an injury. All movement for low back and neck problems must be slow and gentle, to ease into new flexibility and new strength. The specific movements are designed to be used as a preventive program for people who are conscious of the importance of physical fitness. By understanding how our muscles work we can minimize our susceptibility to injury. By improving our bodily alignment we can reduce pain and discomfort. This is especially important during pregnancy, after delivery, or after an injury.

Often my most creative and exciting work is with people who come to me through doctors after surgery, corsets, pills, drugs. They've had all that treatment and it didn't work. By then they're more open to my kind of work. They're at the end of their rope. They've tried everything else. People who are always holding another option, thinking, "I'll just go to the doctor later and get fixed," are the hardest to work with because they're not really listening to you.

Cold packs, heat, massage, corsets, manipulation, pills or injections offer only short term or temporary relief at best. Even after successful surgery people must develop new habits to prevent reinjury. If an exercise program designed to relieve pain is not begun at the first signs of trouble, it becomes increasingly more difficult to reduce or stop the pain. My classes are designed to help develop new habits to last a lifetime.

I work two ways, one way with someone who is really having pain and is unable to function, another way with people who are functioning well. I see many people who have been told to go to bed for two weeks as a remedy for their acute back problems. This suggestion is usually accompanied by a prescription of pain killers and muscle relaxants. Hearing such advice confirms for me that the medical system often does not know how to begin healing back problems. More often than not, at the end of the fourteen days the patient feels little better or worse, and only better until they get out of bed and try to start living again. When you injure your back, it is essential that you begin to learn proper resting positions along with breathing exercises. Our bodies will heal themselves if we direct their movement and make a conscious effort to change our incorrect body habits to proper body movement.

When an injured person is taking pain killers, I ask them to stop because even if they are just turning in bed or shifting positions, on pain killers they can't feel if a movement hurts and they may reinjure themselves without realizing. The pain is a guide. When it is drugged you get to overextend; you get to do more things than your body is ready to have you do. If somebody is in severe pain we do breathing exercises. I tell them if the exercises don't work, take a pill but at least try the breathing. Then maybe they can take only three pills a day instead of four. The first thing I tell people who are able to function is that whenever you're standing up, keep your knees slightly bent. Just that takes about thirty-five percent of the strain off the lower back because the weight of standing gets redistributed to the thigh and belly muscles instead of resting on the vertebrae.

## Breathing

I have people become aware of breathing correctly. As you start to breathe deeply with your diaphragm, and not just in your chest or ribs, you work the lower abdominal muscles which support the spine. There is really no other spinal support system. We have four sets of belly muscles. Three of the four wrap all the way around our spines and they hold it up and dictate our movement. If they are flabby, you can overextend your movement and displace the vertebrae.

People who are out of condition from injury or lack of exercise shouldn't begin a movement program by doing stressful exercises. The first thing they need to develop is the ability to use their belly muscles correctly which means moving their backs. As you lie on the floor and breathe notice how your back moves. As you inhale you can feel your back tend to lift off the floor. When you exhale the back of your waist makes more contact with the floor. Unfortunately, some people have such weak muscles or are so out of tune with their bodies that they can't feel their backs move. Sometimes the muscles are so weakened that full breathing is painful. Is it any wonder, then, that their backs are an open target for injury? I start with relaxing breathing exercises simply to make people aware of what parts move as they breathe, and what parts don't; are they tense across the chest; are they jutting their chin forward or crunching their shoulders?

I also work on the legs to develop calf and thigh muscles with a lot of foot exercises and a lot of ankle and toe movement. Strong, aligned feet are essential. They're what we stand on. I work to develop strong muscles because muscles are meant to bear our body weight and to take the pressure off the joints and bones. If your ankles tilt in when you stand you're usually pulling the sacroiliac joint in your back, and your knee or whole leg is under too much stress. Then we do extension exercises and limber the hip joints.

Traction can be harmful after a back injury. When people hurt themselves, often muscles around the injury become tight and go into spasm because they're protecting that injured area. Those muscles are supposed to stay tight until the area is able to open up and function again. People in this condition should be lying down on their backs with their feet up, knees bent and their heads on pillows depending on the neck condition, or on their sides with a pillow in between their knees and their feet. I start the healing process with breathing and feeling what's happening to try making friends with the body movements that cause pain, so that with full consciousness those movements can be altered or stopped altogether.

My work is different from other approaches which caution you against healing yourself, tell you to listen only to your doctor, and that healing just takes place once a week in the expert's office. Even some chiropractors whose treatments are good may encourage this attitude. If you get into the pattern of having a chiropractor make adjustments for you, but continue your same poor body habits during the week, you won't really heal yourself. I see around a hundred students a week. About seventy of these have seen chiropractors and they're in my class because they have back problems. That makes me question the usefulness of chiropractic for certain conditions. It's better than surgery, of course, but I think it's often too rough or stressful to the injured area. I also have people in my classes who have had back surgery and still have pain. They need gentle exercises plus good breathing.

Basically, I prescribe the same process for all problem conditions. Most back books I've read say it makes a difference whether you have a herniated disc, or a slipped disc, or back strain. I don't think it makes the slightest bit of difference what you have, or why you have it. The healing process requires you to understand what movements aggravate the injured area, and then to avoid reinjury by learning proper basic body mechanics. Learning to feel your balance is what counts. You have to be committed to being kind to yourself. For most people, especially for women, everybody and everything else is more important. People often continue their normal chores with a backache and don't even take rest or exercise breaks. Many people *expect* to be uncomfortable. It's not thought normal to feel really great!

People are healthy who have a good feeling about how they function in life. They're not overwhelmed by living and making their bodies do things for them. I think people who suffer from fatigue or low energy are suffering from ill health. That's *not* how it has to be, even as we get older.

As we get older we have to exercise more. Part of the aging process is that our spinal discs start to dry out. This only tells us how much more we need to move and exercise to keep our circulation going, to keep our bodies supple and strong. We can feel great at any age if we keep ourselves moving, breathing, and, of course, eating well.

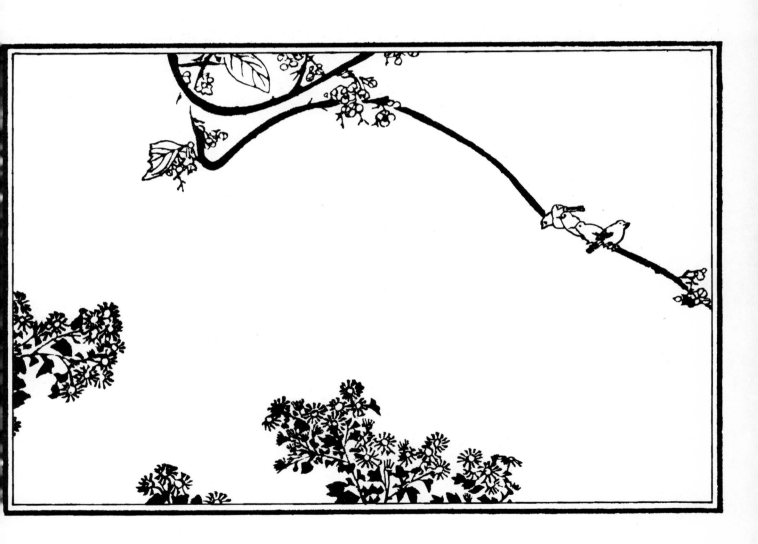

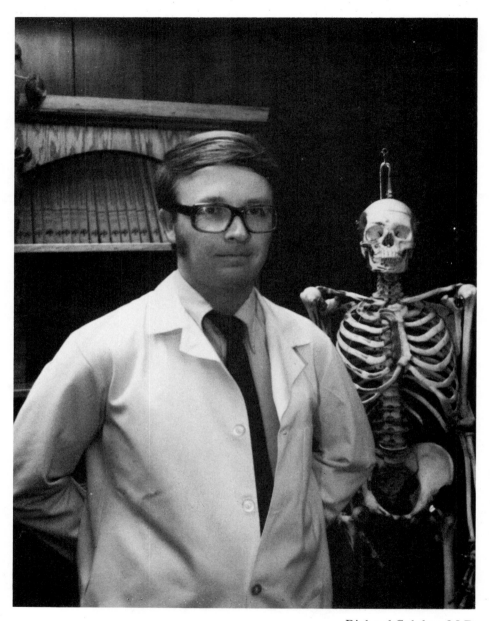

Richard Cobden, M.D.

# An Orthopedic Surgeon: Richard H. Cobden, M.D.

Dr. Richard Cobden is an orthopedic surgeon practicing in California. His work came to my attention through the highest recommendations of friends who had been his patients. I was particularly interested in talking with him because orthopedics is one of the branches of medicine which emphasizes exercise and proper body mechanics as crucial to good health. I interviewed Dr. Cobden in his office in Grass Valley where he has a private practice.

## Diagnosing Your Back Problem

When a patient comes in initially with back pain, it seems as though it might be a very simple thing to tell him, "Yes, you have back pain, and no, it doesn't need surgery. Here are some exercises you should do. Goodbye, we'll see you in two weeks." But we don't really do it that way. We try to take a very carefully detailed history from the patient, to find out how the problem started. We ask the patients to give as much history of its origin as possible. And we talk to them about the process of healing.

We first ask the patient how the problem began. What were the conditions under which it began? Was it an injury or something you just woke up with in the morning? Have there been recent changes in your work habits or lifestyle? Was something else going on at the time, perhaps emotionally or psychologically, that was causing stress? How would you like to feel?

Next we go into how the condition progressed. What happened over the next few days, weeks, or months and what did you do about it? Was it severe enough that you had to quit your job? Did you go to see a physician or decide it was minor enough that you could just 'tough it out'? If you took medication, where did you get it, what type was it, and how often did you take it? Did you use any mechanical methods to relieve the problem such as crutches, a cane, or a corset? Did going to bed bring relief or make the pain worse? What kind of bed do you sleep on? When you sit down, does that make the pain worse or better? Do you have to drive long distances to work and does driving make it better or worse? What are the habits you go through every day? Are you a tidy person who wants to keep everything in the house really neat and clean, or do you let things go? These habits are important because they determine how the patient is going to react to treatment, as well as how well the patient will avoid future exacerbations of the pain.

Then we explore about past history. Did you ever have this sort of a problem before? Years ago did you go through the same situation and then get over it? Did you ever have surgery? Not just on your back, but on any other part of your body? Have you any other current or chronic medical conditions? Are there any areas of overriding concern such as heart disease, high blood pressure or diabetes? We also go over family history for at least two or three generations. Is there anybody in the family who has had anything like what you have now, and is there any chance that it's hereditary?

We try to find out if there are any other symptoms associated with the back problem. How do your eyes and ears work? Do you have any difficulty swallowing? Do you smoke? Do you have troubles with your heart or lungs? Do you have bowel problems? Are you gaining too much weight? When you cough or sneeze does the back pain get worse? Do you find that you trip over your toes occasionally when you walk, or have other motor difficulties? Is running comfortable? Do you have any problem skin condition? Some people with certain severe forms of rheumatoid arthritis, for example, will have a terrible reaction to exposure to sunlight.

After a half an hour of rather intensive questioning and remembering, we go through a physical examination that is at least as exhaustive; and we watch how the patient walks and moves. We talk about movement habits. Can you sit for long periods of time without feeling uncomfortable and having to get up to walk around? We check the patient's reflexes and whether she or he can move the feet, toes and hand synchronously. We check for any lost sensation or motor power. Is there weakness in any of the muscle groups? We check for girth and for length of extremities because sometimes one leg can be a little shorter or longer than the other.

During the course of the examination we observe things of which the patient is often unaware. For example, I might ask you to pick up your socks and shoes. Simply watching how you do that, I can tell a great deal about how you move and get along at home. If you bend over at the waist with your knees straight, I know you don't move very healthily for your back and you'll have continued problems. If you carefully hold on to the table and go down with the knees bent and the back straight, I know you already have some idea about how to move to help heal your back.

Then I might ask a patient to sit up on the table with legs extended. If the patient can do that, I know the problem is not sciatica or a disc problem, but probably a strain. If there is a very tender spot over one or two points in the spine, particularly over the sacroiliac area, and touching or moving that triggers the pain to make it go up and down the spine, or into the legs, then I know the problem is more superficial. It's in the upper ligaments, the muscles or the bursa right under the skin. Those areas respond very well to injections of certain medications and usually one can relieve the pain completely by finding these spots.

After the examination we send you for x-rays if you haven't had them already. X-rays are done for several purposes. Primarily we want to determine whether there's any bone pathology. In older, laboring people, for example, you see tremendous changes: arthritic spurs or collapse of vertebral disc spaces. Sometimes, even in younger people, you'll see what we call spondylolisthesis. This means that there are missing elements in the back which cause it to be unstable. One of the vertebrae may slide forward onto the other, with an action like that of an earthquake fault. When you see a vertebra starting to slide, you know there's going to be trouble because it starts to pinch the nerves in the back.

We also look for congenital anomalies. Sometimes half of the vertebra will be missing or there'll be a tremendous scoliosis that was unsuspected before, or a sacral defect. Once in a while we'll see what is called acute lumbar lordosis, where the sacrum goes out at a ninety degree angle to the spine, actually forming a little shelf out the back. This predisposes the spine to concentrate pressure on the lowest vertebral disc.

We also look for things like tumors. Sometimes the first sign of a cancer appears in the spine and it may show up in backache. In elderly men, particularly, we find that if the prostate forms a cancer, the cancer will metastasize first to the vertebral body. If there's one dense body it will show on the x-ray. Or sometimes a missing piece or a little hole in the bone where there shouldn't be one will show up.

Sometimes we find bone parts missing in a child. I remember one twelve year old boy who was injured in a football game in Southern California about a year before I saw him. He had a lot of pain in the place where he had been struck. A physician saw him soon after the injury and said, "Well, the blow is the cause of it. He'll get over it." In nine hundred and ninety-nine cases out of a thousand, that would be exactly right. In this case, however, it wasn't, because the pain persisted.

The boy had more and more trouble. He couldn't walk or go to school without pain; he was taking aspirin like it was popcorn. The family moved and they finally came to me. I looked him over and thought there was something odd about the boy's problem because the level of his pain was much higher than I expected it should be. We took a series of x-rays of his back. When we were counting the vertebral bodies, we saw that a part of one of them in the midlumbar area was missing. So we did a bone scan on him and it was positive. We sent him to the Sacramento Medical Center where a team of orthopedists, neurosurgeons and pediatric surgeons worked on the boy and removed a giant tumor that was growing on his spine and had begun to close off the cord. Had this thing progressed, he would have been paralyzed within another few weeks. But the tumor was excised completely and the boy made a full recovery. He's back playing football again.

So, we look for lots of things in the x-ray. About ninety-five percent of the time, the x-rays are relatively normal. We don't see anything wrong with the bones, so we assume from that point that the problem is in the muscles, the ligaments or both.

After the x-rays are interpreted, the patient is given instruction on what the condition involves and how he or she should manage it. Most of this instruction is geared to preventing further exacerbations of the same condition, most commonly a lumbosacral, cervical or thoracic strain. The spine works as a unit. Many patients who say their neck or ribs hurt may actually have strained their lower backs. We have to treat the entire spine, the entire body, in fact. If the patient, for example, is five foot four inches tall and weighs two hundred and eighty pounds, what has to be done is pretty obvious. We talk about proper diet, getting muscle tone back and developing good health habits.

The hardest thing I have to convince my patients of is the need to stay in bed for two or three weeks after they've had an acute back strain. They just don't want to do it. Two or three weeks in bed to them is like ten years in San Quentin. Time after time, I'll send them home with instructions to stay in bed, and they'll come back in a week and say, 'It's not getting better. You've got to do something.' So I put them in the hospital, put them to bed for another week, and they get better. I'll ask, 'Why did you get better here and not at home?' It turns out that when the phone rang, they got up to answer it. They went out to use the bathroom, took a shower, made dinner, watered the garden. You begin to discover that bed rest at home is rarely bed rest at all.

The problems people run into with back pain are generally caused by incorrect body mechanics. If you thoroughly understand body mechanics, you probably will never get into trouble with your back. If trouble does occur, one should understand the need for rest first, and then the need for exercise after the period of pain has gone by.

## Penny Pinching Exercise

If the patient bends over from the waist with the knees straight, I explain how to bend at the knees, how to keep the back straight and how to concentrate on good body mechanics. Even the simplest action, such as brushing your teeth in the morning, can be a tremendous strain on the back if while doing it you lean forward at the waist with your knees straight. So we teach people little tricks, like opening the cabinet below the sink and resting your foot on it while you brush. That takes the strain off the back. For people who tend to lordosis, a sway back, pot belly and poor posture, we suggest a simple exercise. In fact, we give this to almost all the patients. It's called the Goldthwaite exercise. Doctor Goldthwaite was a famous orthopedic surgeon in New York who was trying to find an exercise for back patients who couldn't handle a complicated routine. There were too many exercises being offered and the patients simply could not absorb everything they were being taught. Goldthwaite tried to think of one exercise that would benefit them as much and as continuously as possible.

The exercise he devised is known as penny pinching. To do it, the patient stands still, heels together and toes a little bit apart, pretending he or she has a penny caught in the crack of the buttocks, in the gluteal fold. You push the gluteal muscles, that is, the buttocks together as hard as you can, to hold onto the penny and do it frequently. When you try that exercise, you find that your back muscles begin to straighten up, your abdominal muscles pull in, your pelvis tilts forward and your entire spine aligns itself over your heels. Fashion models seem to use this technique when they are standing for proper posture. We tell patients with poor posture to do this continuously. And it works!

## Physical Therapy

We find that Williams' exercises, traditional exercises for strengthening the abdominal muscles and stretching the back are helpful too. If the patients need more intensive exercise then we'll send them to physical therapy. The physical therapist will then give them additional methods such as working on a stationary bicycle, swimming exercises, stretching and other postures, and perhaps reducing exercises.

If patients come in who are unable to do exercises due to a heart condition, muscular disease, or severe pain, we give them a support garment. This may be a corset, a very small back brace, or a device called a criss cross brace which is basically a large piece of velcro that folds in front and holds in the abdomen. We find that if the abdominal muscles are protected and in good shape, they will support half the weight of the body, allowing the back to rest. Corsets, girdles and back braces are like crutches. They will usually prevent pain during the acute phase, but they are no means to prevent future back pain. For that reason, we always tell patients to stop using these devices and begin developing their own muscles once their back pain is relatively alleviated.

Long term prevention is emphasized at this point so that the patients understand they will have to be their own therapists for the rest of their lives. This means getting the weight down perhaps, building the muscles up, watching body mechanics very carefully and thoroughly understanding what their specific back condition is and how to prevent problems in the future. Most patients will listen and follow these instructions and so will stay out of trouble.

But quite a few people quit doing exercises instead of continuing them for prevention. After two or three years free of pain, they may slip back into the old bad habits. You can visualize the spine as being like a stack of coins. It's extremely stable when it's vertical, but the moment you tilt it and load it, it becomes unstable and starts to fall apart. If people understand the structure of their backs in those terms, it's unlikely that they're going to get into problem situations by moving incorrectly. The things that we teach people about body mechanics like exercise and physical fitness, have to become a lifelong program.

## Resistance To Getting Well

About ten or fifteen percent of the patients will keep coming back with the same problems. They usually fall into two categories: either they are patients who for some reason, don't want to get better and know it; or they have an unconscious psychological fear which prevents them from getting well. The reasons may be complicated or simple. If there is litigation going on, a lawsuit, a Worker's Compensation claim or if for some reason the patient doesn't feel confident enough psychologically or physically to return to work, their pain will continue. Whether they are aware of this or not, I can't always say. I haven't often seen patients who I thought were deliberately lying about their back pain. Once or twice, I've been fooled. I had an insurance man come in one day to show me a film, taken through the bushes, of a patient he had been observing. This patient had been complaining of back pain for about a year. The film showed the patient picking up a heavy tire he had changed on his truck, then carrying two large tarpaper rolls up a ladder and laying them on his roof. This patient had told me that he couldn't pick up his shoes. It was obvious that the guy had fooled me; but that was such an exception that I can remember it out of all my cases in the last five years. I don't think there are many like that.

There are patients who, for one reason or another, will not want to get better and there's not much you can do about it. You just carry them along. Often, they are easy to identify because they will resist further treatment. If you suggest they see a neurosurgeon, for example, or someone who might operate on them, they will usually be reluctant and refuse because they want to preserve the status quo. They are in the minority and probably represent only about two percent of all the patients with back pain.

Another category is that of the patient who really has a problem, like a protruded disc or perhaps even a tumor, or something else that is relatively disastrous, who isn't responding to treatment and yet doesn't want any further treatment at all. He is either afraid of it, having had a bad experience before, or just doesn't trust it. The patient who is grossly obese and just can't make up his or her mind to lose the weight and get back to a normal state also falls in this category. These are tough patients to deal with, the ones no one seems to be able to help. You can nurse them through a difficult period but they are likely to be back again and again and to need hospitalization many times. Mainly they are people who are overweight or people who don't exercise or watch their body mechanics. There are reasons why they won't do these things, but I can't quite fathom all of them.

Sometimes these people need psychiatric or psychological help, or they may need family counseling because they are under outside stress. They respond to the stress by becoming overweight or by not cooperating with the rehabilitation program and, consequently, they get into physical trouble. Their physical trouble is the reason we end up seeing them. It's like holding onto a tiger's tail. You've got one problem in your hand but there is another problem at the other end and you can't get near it. This sort of person may represent one to two percent of the patients. The other ninety-five percent of people with back problems will be better, one way or the other.

There are some people who have a minor back problem but refuse to do preventive exercises until the problem becomes severe. Again, you're talking about psychological considerations. What is that person's makeup? What makes him decide to do that? Is he a macho type who is just not going to pay attention to minor problems because he thinks he's so tough that he can handle anything? Or is he so burdened by other worries that a back ache seems minor to him until it does become a major problem?

People sometimes want to be sick. A person might wish to be sick to be able to say to his antagonists, 'See what you've done to me. Now you're going to have to take care of me.' That situation does happen. You can usually spot people who have a great need to be disabled in order to get out of stressful situations. For instance, the patient who deliberately jumps on a motorcycle without a helmet on a rainy day and goes riding down the road at a hundred miles an hour. There's some kind of a wish to get hurt going on in that man's mind. There has to be! I can't conceive of anybody deliberately doing such dangerous things otherwise.

Once in a while I run across people who do have a need to be disabled, and if you treat their disability too successfully you're in trouble. I remember one spectacular example, a patient who had had a chronic ulcer for ten years. He had not responded to treatment and had consistently refused surgery. Surgery is the last hope for ulcer disease. After you've tried all the conservative therapies, medicine hasn't anything left to offer but to take the stomach out. Finally under the strong urging of his family, this patient agreed to surgery. The surgery was successful but about two weeks afterward, when he realized it was in fact successful, he went stark raving mad. For the next two years he was in a mental hospital, because he had realized he didn't have a disability any more. So we shouldn't assume that everybody wants to be well. In cases like that, if you can preserve a little bit of the disability, or at least the thought of it, you may be better off than curing it altogether. That is an uncommon situation but we have to be aware of the possibility. In this sort of situation, a psychiatrist may be helpful. But psychiatrists are no help at all to a patient who doesn't want counseling. Somehow you have to get people to the point where they can understand what they need. Failing that, you would just leave a minimum disability so that the person has a psychological crutch, but is well enough to function and to feel that he or she is a fairly whole human being.

It's not really helpful to tell the people involved what my opinion is in those situations. If you tell the family, they just get mad. If you tell a patient, he says, 'You're a liar; you got me all misunderstood.' There is no better way to make a patient angry than to tell the complete truth in a situation where it's not wanted. So you have to assess each situation individually. But again, that's an unusual situation. Most patients want to know what's wrong with them, and most of them deal with it very well.

## Learning Preventive Care

Many people fall into the category of simply not being able to get into the habit, being too busy, or not really believing that exercise will work. There's little in our environment today that supports self-healing or preventive medicine. You may be fighting the schedule of your job which doesn't give you time to stop for a couple of exercises during the day. You're fighting your doubts that exercise has much to do with mental and physical balance. These attitudes are changing and it's becoming more common to do sports like tennis or running. We're becoming aware now of other cultures which emphasize physical fitness. In Germany, in East Germany particularly, in the last ten or fifteen years, there's widespread participation in physical fitness programs, even before people start school. In China many people take breaks from work to do exercise routines during the day. This practice is also widespread in Japan. I think the time will come when we'll do that here in the United States, but it's still very difficult to convince patients to devote a certain amount of time each day to exercise. The resistance level is high.

With most of those patients, I give one definite exercise to do at a definite time. The Goldthwaite exercise is something that can be done easily all day long. It becomes second nature.

## Depression and Exercise

Once in a while, I'll come across a patient whom I cannot definitely diagnose. Their back hurts; their legs hurt; their joints ache; their eyeballs hurt; everything hurts and they want to know what's wrong. We run exhaustive tests and x-rays and we can't find anything out of order. Generally these people appear to be a bit depressed and upset at themselves. I will put them on a strict regime of exercise. They may bicycle twenty minutes a day up steep hills, swim fifty laps every day, do twenty-five pushups in the morning before they even get dressed. I have them write it all down on a list each day, and come in every two weeks to show me they've done it. If you put these patients on a good diet, give them good exercises, and get them out of bad habits, like smoking or drinking too much, they almost invariably start feeling a lot better. They say, 'All right, now someone's told me what to do. By golly, I'm going to do it.' They feel better physically, and because of their accomplishments they start to feel better about themselves psychologically.

## Backs of Different Ages

In orthopedic medicine there are different treatments for different age groups. If a very young patient has back pain, we proceed much differently than we would if she or he were middle-aged or elderly because young people don't often get back pain. When they do, there is usually something seriously wrong. A two or three year old child, for example, who has back pain is presumed to have an infection in the disc space or a tumor until proven otherwise. Such infections are very serious in children and can be fatal. So you have to work fast to get the infection relieved, treated, drained, administer the proper antibiotics and do whatever else has to be done.

In cases of teenaged or subteen back pain we also look for serious causes. In their age group, the incidence of tumor goes way up because they are growing rapidly. An embryonic tumor that's been sitting around since they were born can suddenly explode and start to grow. Sometimes, the cause can be a protruded disc or it can be a problem of trauma. Accidents where teenagers fall off their motorbikes and break their backs are unfortunately quite common. Or kids dive into a river, break their necks, and end up quadriplegic. We treat a lot of accident cases with teenagers.

We begin to see strain conditions such as disc problems and sciatica in the middle twenties to thirties age group. People who get them are usually young working people who are quite vigorous and need to keep working, so you have to treat them a bit differently. The approach to the twenty to thirty age group is to try to relieve their pain and get them back in working condition as quickly as possible because of their overriding concern to keep food on the table or take care of the family.

In the forty-five to sixty year old group, you run into problems of degeneration. People at that age are usually no longer fit; they are beginning to lose their muscle tone; their problems with body mechanics become prominent. With them you have to concentrate on an exercise and rehabilitation routine and proper nutrition.

In the sixty to eighty year old group, you begin to get into some of the more severe degenerative diseases. Problems of degenerative arthritis with osteoporosis is five to ten times more prevalent in women of that age than in men. Osteoporosis means a loss of bone substance and usually occurs about five to ten years after menopause, probably due to rapid hormonal changes. It is characterized by thinning of the bone. Thus bones become susceptible to fractures and injury and begin to compress. When you see older people with hump backs, 'the Dowager's hump,' what you are really seeing is multiple compression fractures of the upper thoracic vertebrae. If you took an x-ray, you would see that each of their vertebrae, instead of being nice and square, was wedge shaped. They start to slump forward more and more. These problems can be dealt with by restoring the calcium, phosphorus, and in some cases the flouride to their systems in order to harden the bone. Also we may brace them so that they will straighten up and begin to get the proper posture again. In the older age group, we again look for incidence of tumor. Tumors appear in the very young and the very old. We look for prostatic tumor and for breast tumor. If these start to metastasize, it shows up in the spine first. We look for the cause of pain in the back and sometimes find a tumor that's migrated from somewhere else in the body. Primary tumors of the spine are very rare.

## Medicine Today

One challenge that faces a lot of us today in medicine is that we can't rely on our credentialed authority any more. It used to be that doctors would tell a patient to do something and that was it; you didn't question it; you just went out and did it. Now patients want to know why you're telling them to do something; they want full explanations, and they want to be able to make their own decisions. Sometimes, complete explanations are hard to give. If you tell them that it's psychological, then you'll probably turn them off. But a lot of medicine is psychological. A lot of traditional Western medicine is psychological. Most doctors sixty or one hundred years ago didn't know scientifically what they were doing, but the patients thought they did, and that helped. I think a lot of any medicine is psychological. If you have a really positive attitude about recovering from an illness, you will probably get better.

Health is what each individual perceives as his or her most comfortable state of existence. I am stating it as it pertains to the individual because I think health to one person is not health to another. I hesitate to define health as 'the absence of disease,' as Western medicine used to, because that doesn't seem to mean very much; it sounds too neutral. Health is a person's positive feeling of well-being.

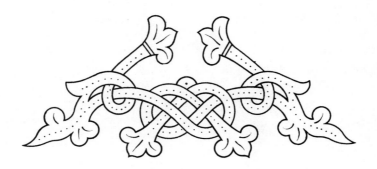

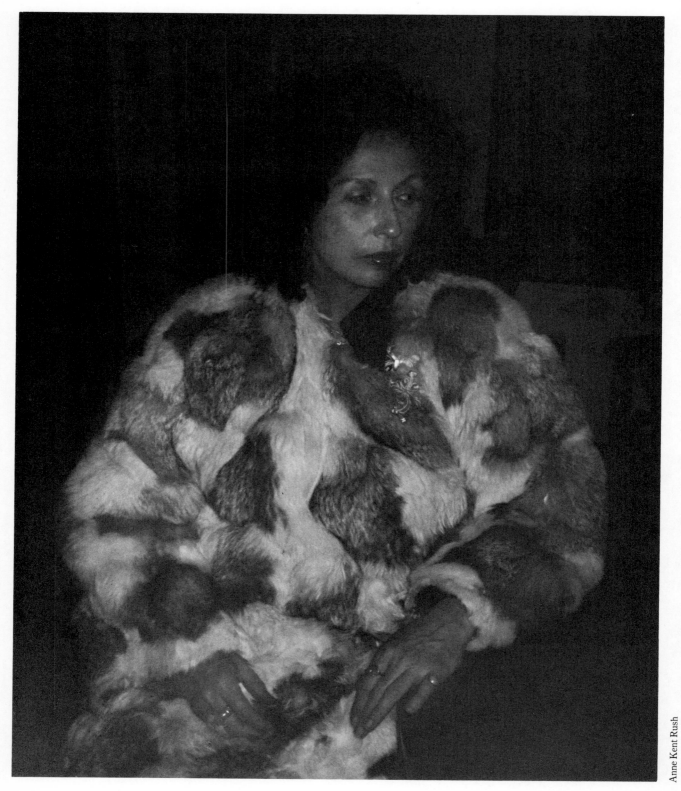

Anne Kent Rush

Dr. Evon Karanoff

# An Acupuncturist: Dr. Evon Karanoff

Acupuncture is a whole system of Oriental medicine based on the theory that health is gained through the free flow of chi, or electromagnetic energy currents in the body. Acupuncture points are centers of chi energy. Tiny needles are often used in acupuncture treatments, inserted into the patient's skin on the specific chi points corresponding to the problem.

Evon Karanoff studied acupuncture in Asia and in Europe, principally in France, and returned to the U.S. to open her practice in Berkeley, California. She has been trained in allopathic medicine, Tibetan medicine, western and Chinese herbalism, homeopathy, classic Chinese acupuncture, Ryodoraku, French techniques according to Soulie de Mourant and auricular (ear acupuncture) techniques under Dr. Nogier. Karanoff also teaches privately.

## Acupuncture and the Back

Many people know little about acupuncture even today. They often don't understand it is a complete system of medicine for all problems. And if they hear about it often they worry about the use of needles. Ninety-eight percent of all acupuncture is completely painless. There may be some sensation of pain if the client has a lot of tension or energy. But when I confront a great knot under the skin I'm not going to go in with the needle. I'll soften it with herbs and massage. I'll do all kinds of things to loosen it in order to make that part of the body receptive. I won't fight with it. The use of force is the main cause of pain. But it is not necessary. There is basic energy in the body. If there has been blockage of that energy, in your leg or foot, for example, it feels as if your foot has gone to sleep. When the energy and circulation return to these areas, there are many kinds of subtle sensation, but rarely pain. Some people feel the energy as tingling, sometimes itching. Others feel a sort of tickling or numbness. One's response to the release of tension is very subjective. Often it's felt neither as pain nor as pleasure but simply as sensation.

Statistics have shown that acupuncture is highly effective in treating any form of paralysis. It's also been shown to be highly effective in relieving rheumatoid arthritis. Arthritis, more than the other problems requires a careful regimen of diet and herbal supplements.

A book on acupuncture that I'd recommend for beginners is Steven Palos' THE CHINESE ART OF HEALING. He's an excellent acupuncturist and presents a good overview of the principles involved in acupuncture and in breathing therapy. Acupuncture is only one section of Chinese medicine. Traditionally, it is comprised of special breathing and meditation techniques, and the use of herbs and exercises. The classics said if all you do is take the symptoms away you are an inferior doctor; you should treat the whole person. Heeding this, I may send my patients to other specialists to complement my work.

Acupuncture, very simply, is the assistance of the movement of 'chi' or energy in the body. The philosophy behind it is very old. It's called Taoism because that's the historical name of the philosophy, but it actually predates what we think of as Taoism. The earliest book on the philosophy is approximately four thousand years old, and it refers to 'the ancient classics'! The system deals with rivers of energy in the body. If there is dysfunction in the body it means that an energy river is blocked, or dammed by a material that the Chinese call 'rough matter.' Rough matter is unexpelled waste material that can solidify into a kind of gristle. Or it can calcify and deposit around the bones, as in arthritis. Such a deposit then blocks the path of the chi or energy streams.

The purpose of performing acupuncture is to increase the flow of chi which breaks the circulation barriers. Then the body must be encouraged to eliminate the waste matter and re-establish its balanced energy pattern. If you let the rough matter accumulate over time, you begin to get products of secondary blockage like cellulite or cancer. It's important to be sensitive to your own tension so you can clear energy blocks early and prevent serious problems. You don't have to be an acupuncturist to know when something is a little strange, or when something's going really well.

The ancient practice of acupuncture was based on having the client come for a checkup once or twice a year to make sure everything was all right and to correct imbalances before they became dysfunctional. The tradition in ancient China was that if the physician kept the person well, she or he was paid. If the patient became ill, then the doctor forfeited the money. It's really a strange situation for me as an acupuncturist to treat people who come to me after they're very ill or have had four operations. Those kinds of cases aren't even in the books because acupuncture is a preventive system. So a lot of my work is developmental.

I once had a patient who had had a lamenectomy, a surgical fusion of the nerves of the spine to the vertebrae. When he first came to me, I said, 'There's nothing I can do for a case like yours. It isn't in the acupuncture books. All I can do is help you feel better, and that will require constant maintenance.' He worked very hard at it. He did everything I told him. His diet was strict. It took us two years to achieve, but he did have great recovery. Some people have the notion that they can come, have a needle put in, and everything in their lives will be solved. It doesn't always work that way. Sometimes it does, not always. There have been remarkable cases, cases where I would not have expected any results. A lot of the healing depends on the participation of the person who comes. Hopefully you start treatments before their condition becomes advanced or severe.

The conditions I treat vary a lot. Chinese acupuncture recognizes that most diseases are seasonal. At the solstice and at the equinox there will be enormous influxes of the diseases particular to those seasons. In the fall I often see people with lung diseases. Kidney diseases prevail in winter. There are, of course, many variations. It doesn't necessarily mean that only the specific organ is not working right. The kidneys, for instance, affect the chemical balance of the blood, so you'll have more kidney related diseases like arthritis in the winter.

There are periods when all I seem to do is deal with back problems. I find inevitably that difficulty in the back will be concentrated in the pelvic area. There's always a slight pelvic twist and when that is corrected, the spine falls into line. The pelvis is a chalice of power in the body. The hara, or energy center, is in the lower abdomen, and it's cradled by the pelvic bowl. The whole pelvis is also an area that responds immediately to fear. There's a direct psychological connection between our early toilet training, our sensual and sexual prohibitions, and the twisting of the pelvis. Whenever the individual gets stressed and starts reacting in his or her habitual patterns of fear, the pelvis tenses again and is usually held off balance. Then the whole back is forced to compensate for the twist in its foundation. The imbalance goes all the way up the spine until finally even the neck becomes stiff. Often people come in with bursitis or a stiff neck, and I find that what's wrong with them is a pelvis out of line. You may take the pain away from the upper back but unless this whole fundamental alignment is balanced, the pains will recur.

Acupuncture, by working on energy patterns, activates and relaxes the musculature and its surrounding nervous system. It also influences the balance of secretions in various parts of the body, even in the brain. Not only does the pain leave after acupuncture but habit patterns are also largely released. Then the initial response is available to change. Often if people go to a practitioner who works on the superficial musculature or the bones, the habit which caused their problem isn't broken and they have to keep going back. Acupuncture gets at the root of the imbalance and thus is often a quicker treatment than others.

There are many important acupuncture points in the back. Along the sides of the vertebrae are points that we call U-points. They are important in acupuncture because they make direct connections with the body's organs. Through treating the U-points you not only treat the back itself but also the organs that are connected to each point. Very often somebody with a serious back problem will have a sluggish liver or an enlarged spleen. Inevitably their back pain is governed by the point which corresponds to the affected organ.

I base my practice on the Oriental system. I'm a classic acupuncturist in my philosophy

In my practice, of course, I use what's available. If somebody needs a Western treatment such as surgery, for instance, or anything else that could help, I recommend it. But my basic premises are classic Oriental ones.

Emotional problems often correspond to back problems. The back is where many people hold tension and psychological stress. 'Feeling your back is to the wall,' for instance. But to work on the back exclusively is counter-productive because stress is a slippery thing. It will slide around from one place in the body to the other. In dealing with a back problem, I treat the whole body, and the whole psyche. People of different ages are treated in slightly different ways. For instance you don't usually use needles on a person younger than five or seven years. You usually don't need them, for one thing. Children are very soft, you know. Their patterns aren't as hardened as ours. The problem is the parents usually; they need the needles! But I've treated children's back problems with finger pressure on the points. Acupuncture invades the body. So it shouldn't be used on people in vulnerable conditions: young children, people who are extremely weak or extremely old, or women who are pregnant.

Since I began work in this field I haven't been ill. Before that, I was always dealing with some ailment. In order to be healthy, people need vision, a commitment. The obstacles that prevent this are the things that make us ill. It's often our own willingness

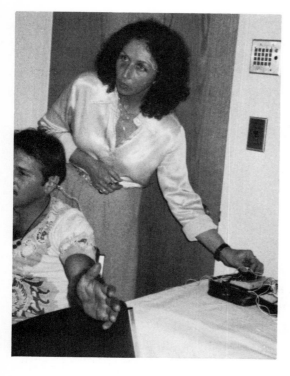

Research in thermography and auricular acupuncture at Parnassus

to live in chains that make us ill. The world can be a strange and terrifying place. When we're born we're very vulnerable. Parents unconsciously offer food and protection in exchange for their child's freedom. This is called civilization and acculturation. Then people grow up with the unrecognized agreement that they must barter freedom for existence. The choice is offered again and again and it seizes our life, and takes our space. We often can't accept freedom because in the back of our minds is an unrecognized belief that if we do, we are violating our agreement and we will die. This outdated and ineffectual security blanket that we carry around is the basis of all neurosis. We have to let it go in layers gradually to become more fully functional. One is free to the degree one has managed to shake loose the attachment to false security.

We need to align our rhythms with the rhythm of the planets and of the earth. That is what we call being in tune, or being in flow. There are rules in Chinese medicine for observing these rhythms but few people these days have the time or opportunity to practice them fully.

I don't think of health as something one achieves. It's a natural state. It's our heritage. It is the nature of being. The thrust of the organism, as I see it, is to life. So it's not a matter of doing something new to get healthy. It's a matter of letting go of the things that make one ill. The single most effective health giving measure I can think of is to become free, and you can do this slowly through the observance of your own body rhythms as expressions of your deepest self.

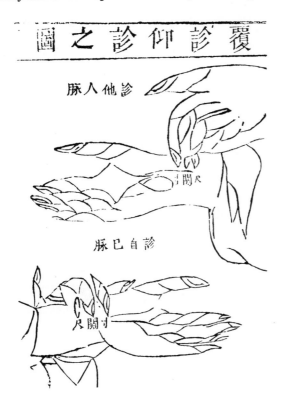

Instructions for pulse taking, from *T'u Chu Mo Chueh* by Chang Shih-hsien, Ming period.

Erika Asher

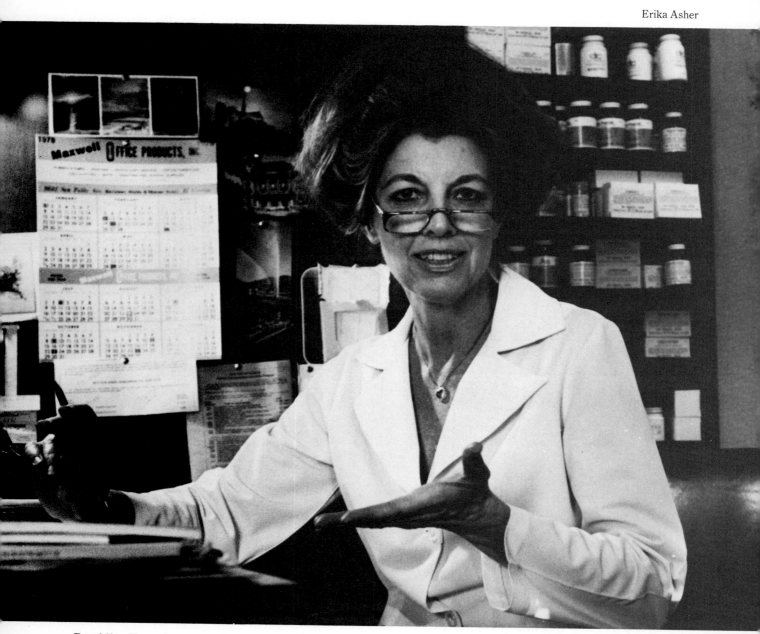

Dr. Alice Francis

# A Chiropractor: Dr. Alice Francis

Chiropractic is a system of medicine based on the belief that health is largely maintained by proper stimulation of the nerves branching from the spinal cord to the rest of the body, and by balanced nutrition. The practice of chiropractic includes movement of the patient's spine by the doctor. Alice Francis was born in Oakland and has been a chiropractor in California for thirty years. Dr. Francis also has a specialty in nutrition.

When I was sixteen, I was going to a chiropractor as a patient and he said, "Why don't you go to chiropractic college?" In the summertime I had worked a bit in his office and enjoyed it very much. He was a professor at the school. I started my studies, and I became the youngest graduate ever in the state of California, before I was twenty-one. The school was fine and boasted a free clinic. It was in downtown Oakland in the Tapscott Building and we had the Corpango Mortuary as one of our laboratories. We would go there to dissect the bodies of people who had died of diseases we needed to study. We studied the muscles and the full line up of nerves in the body.

When I came out of the school I went right into practice with a man about fifty years old who had been a chiropractic doctor during the war years in the forties. He was also a general practitioner. He delivered babies, made house calls and gave first aid treatment. A chiropractor is not licensed to use injections or pain killers, so his patients really had to have some tolerance for pain. But there was such a shortage of medical help then that it was wonderful that he lived in an area where he could go ahead and be of service. I worked with him for nine years and our practice was the broadest practice that I can imagine, from psychiatric cases to delivering babies, from accident cases to skin diseases and taking care of infants.

## Nutrition

Since then my practice has been more limited to nutrition and chiropractic. We deal with people who come in with a pain in their backs, their necks, their legs. It is up to me to decide whether that pain is skeletal or caused by an internal organ. I've done chiropractic work along with work on nutrition. For the past twenty years nutrition has been one of my mainstays. My daughter contracted cancer when she was a small child. So I went into nutrition because I didn't want her subjected to any type of destructive chemotherapy or radiation. She's twenty-two now, and a mother of two children. She did have to have surgery and she survived, and she's doing well. I treated her with vitamins, minerals and enzymes.

Enzymes are some of the main correctives that can be used to treat cancer. Cancer is a metabolic disorder. If the body's metabolism is off balance, the cells receive ill-digested food. That inferior food makes inferior tissues, and could cause tumor growth and other abnormalities in the tissues themselves. A person may get a skin eruption which won't heal because the proper nutrients aren't available in the body. So we must go back to nutrition and metabolism. In a case like my daughter's, there was a predisposition to cancer. Because she has a weak pancreas and a weak liver she might develop cancer anywhere in her body at any time. She's had leukemia twice. She had to learn to live for health first, in order to reap the reward of living a full and vital life. But she does well, and it isn't a bad life. It's one that's free from foods that are refined, which is how everyone should live anyway.

If people would just live in the way we were made to live—on whole, unadulterated foods—and use meat only sparingly to season our vegetable dishes we would do well. I maintain that the people in nations that are the biggest meat eaters are the most barbaric. Usually people we "civilized" cultures might label "savages" are very docile. They're mostly grain eaters, sweet potato eaters, banana eaters and they're more docile than those civilized nations that wage war and kill for greed. I studied nutrition in San Francisco under Dr. Ernst Krebs. He was the discoverer of pangamic acid, $B^{15}$. He has worked for many years with Laetrile as well, which is vitamin $B^{17}$. The use of these vitamins in treating arthritis and cancer is the subject of a political controversy here in the United States.

I prescribe nutrition treatments in the forms of tablets or capsules, powders and liquids. For instance, enzymes would very rarely be prescribed in liquid form. They would almost always be taken in tablets with a meal to aid a particular gland. If the pancreas needed treatment, we'd give pancreatic enzymes. Sometimes I like to give whole, freeze-dried, powdered, pancreas because that way no intrinsic part of the organ is left out.

Over the past seventy-five years, we have found that blood has many more properties and constituents than were recognized earlier. Actually those constituents were there all the time, but we didn't know it. So I use that same premise for nutritional analysis when I treat a patient. If I give whole freeze-dried powdered pancreas substance, I'm not missing anything. If something useful as an anticancer therapy is later discovered to be in the organ, I've been giving it for years. So I look for certain houses like Standard Brands and Pickrell that put out whole organic substances.

I'm happy to say, we have quite a few hours of nutrition training in the chiropractic study which is an important difference between it and medical training. I went to daily classes in nutrition and biochemistry for one year. Then I've had to enlarge upon every-thing I learned there because the amount of information has mushroomed. Thirty years ago I used to think along the lines of giving a person certain foods to eat plus supple-mental vitamins, minerals and enzymes. Now I think of megadoses. I learned most about nutrition from studying diet. But therapy is a different thing. You go beyond maintenance to correction. Vitamin A can help a person's skin stay smooth, but suppose they get a rash all over their body. They could eat foods rich in vitamin A from now on without curing their rash. They need a megadose of vitamins for a cure.

## Chiropractic Manipulation

In my practice I have a partner who is a darling great-grandfather. He's the same man I came out of college to work with. He's eighty-three years old now. His name is Dr. Edward A. Ogden. Of all the chiropractors in the Bay Area today, I think he and I are the closest in our approaches to health. We look at a person, and listen to them well when they come in. The interview and the history are important to us. We always give a chiropractic adjustment if the patient will accept it. But that isn't usually our only thrust. Most often it is chiropractic plus nutrition.

Chiropractic teaches the maintenance of health through the stimulation of all the nerves as they leave the spinal cord, and the feeding of the body to maintain a level of both psychological and physical health. It's stimulating to the metabolism and the nervous energies that are always present in the human body. When I consider health, I think of the systems that are in the body and whether they maintain the body at peak performance level. My approach is three fold. I may use cleansing also. A patient who has arthritis is affected by a disease because the system is dirty. Waste materials are being deposited in all the joints. The toxic buildup from the body's metabolism is filtering in, and they're developing enlarged joints while their blood vessels are narrowing. So I would need to prescribe a cleansing. Chiropractic deals with cleansing of the tissues, the adequate elim-ination of toxins so the metabolism is at its peak and all systems perform well.

I think chiropractic has always been presented in the schools as a preventive system. I want my patients to feel better when they leave the office right away, and to maintain their well being and resistance to disease. I think all chiropractors do.

Contracted, feverish muscles pull bones out of articulation to varying degrees. When I make a spinal adjustment, I'm suggesting to the tight muscle, "Release. Relax." And it may let go completely or only partially. Then I may massage it out a bit more. I don't look like I give rough adjustments, do I? If it doesn't let go this time, I'll see the patient in a day or a week and make an adjustment then. I put hot packs on the patient's back for twenty minutes. The packs are made of a clay and dropped in a solution which keeps them hot. We wrap the clay packs in Turkish towels, and we put the steamy heated packs on the whole length of your spine as you lie on the table. You're told to rest and enjoy the heat.

I also use shiatsu pressure point treatments on the spine, the face, the abdomen and the bottom of the feet. If a person comes to me with a severe case of sciatic neuritis, where the nerve trunk and the nerve endings are sore clear down the back of the leg into the foot, I will work on the feet first with massage. Then I work up the leg to the back. I counsel the patient to sit up once an hour, straight, take a deep breath, and sit well back in the chair with both feet flat on the floor. I give people exercises to do every day once every hour, and it keeps them thinking about body health.

## Sleep

We also talk about sleep and sleep surfaces. Water beds are not good. I will admit though that when my husband and I take a trip, we usually try to find a water bed in a hotel or motel somewhere, just for a change, just for fun so we can say we've gone on a vacation. But we don't own one. We have a hard, firm mattress. That's what's best for a back. The back needs support. The firmer the bed the better. In fact, some people with enough padding on their bones could sleep on the floor. If your back is very sore, and you don't have a good bed, I would recommend sleeping on the floor on a couple of folded up blankets. Lie flat without a pillow. Get the tension on your spine equalized on either side of the body. Sometimes you have such a sore back that you wouldn't want to lie flat on one hip because of the pain. But it will gradaully ease up, especially if you're on a cleansing diet, drinking some carrot or grapefruit juice and eating light. I like to suggest that people sleep without a pillow, at least for an hour morning and night. If the neck is sore, I suggest an electric heating pad turned on low rolled under the neck, actually hugging it. The spine and the head should be on the same plane. This helps the body to normalize its spinal alignment. Another cause of poor sleep is an elevation of sugar in the blood. In our society we've put sugar everywhere. You can read it on the labels of prepared foods. Unfortunately we're over-sugared in this country.

The vitamin tryptophane seems to feed the sleep center in the brain. You can give tryptophane for maybe two to three weeks, and some insomniacs respond. The person who doesn't respond to tryptophane might benefit from the herb valerian root. Valerian comes in a couple of forms. One is a tea and they might drink that at bedtime or during the day to relax and calm themselves, or they can take it in one or two tablets before going to bed at night. Valerian is also used for blood pressure control for the person who is always anxious, who sees every situation as a stressful one. The "Oh dear, I'm late for lunch. I wonder if they'll have anything left?" type. Rather than being kind to themselves and saying, "I'm glad I'm late. It will be quiet and I can take longer to eat", some people always take the anxious approach. That sort of person I usually treat with valerian root, which is a beneficial herb that works wonderfully.

There are certain vitamins and minerals that are used by bones and joints which can be helpful to people with arthritis and a history of back pain. There is B15 pangamic acid. Because of the controversy surrounding its use, B15 has been a controversial vitamin and it goes on the market and off at the whim of the politicians. For instance, people sometimes have to go to Mexico for it. I use it extensively. It's beneficial in one-half to one-third of the cases. And for those, it's the only answer. Those cases are usually problems of inflammation: arthritis and joint problems where little lumps might be developing in their joints, or a hump and stiffness in their neck.

Many people who've had other prior treatments—surgery, laminectomies, disc operations, traction, back brace—come to me. They run the full gamut of treatment and still feel bad. They say, "I am coming to you as a last resort. I'm on permanent disability. I can't survive the way I am." I overturn their way of life. I have them cut down on the amount of meat they eat. I have them increase the amount of vegetables they eat. Sometimes I have them fast twelve hours a day to let their bodies rest. I take them off coffee. I give them an exercise to use to learn how to stand and sit upright. I give them vitamins, minerals, digestives, and treatments each week for three weeks or so.

## Many Causes

Their problems may clear up entirely, in spite of the failure of the previous treatments. And I think the reason for this is that perhaps their maladies had more than one cause. Perhaps in addition to a back strain or a slipped vertebra, they also had a kidney inflammation, or poorly functioning kidneys. So having a back operation wouldn't take care of the whole person. Therefore, I consider myself a general practitioner, using a holistic approach.

When I see a patient with a backache, I think about their bones, but I also think about their kidneys and their gall bladders, or constipation. If it's an older person, I think about menopause and its depletion of the body's hormone system. I take all those things into consideration when I see a person with a back problem. I treat a very broad spectrum. When they come in with a back ache I may in fact wind up treating the effects of menopause, and so their back gets better.

## Exercises

I always tell people with back problems to stand tall in the morning; to stretch toward the ceiling with their fingertips, stretch up off the heels onto the toes, then to come back onto the heels and lean forward over to the floor without bending the knees much, then stand with the feet apart and then reach one hand down towards the opposite foot, and the other hand over to the other foot, then stand up and reach to the ceiling taking a deep breath. I tell them to do this maybe three times, near a window so some oxygen comes into the lungs. And, if they feel like it, they can jog for a minute or two. Starting the morning this way has made me feel good. And each day I drink an eight ounce glass of hot water with the juice of half a fresh lemon in it to wash out my stomach and get the elimination started in my body. I don't eat for at least half an hour afterwards.

People should sit close to the table with both feet on the floor. When people hunch over to eat, they don't digest as well. When a person has back trouble, s/he has it sitting, sleeping and driving. Most of it is due to poor posture. Car seats today have you partially lying down while driving. You don't sit upright like a truck driver does. We don't have that much ease in the seats of our cars. We sit too tilted back so that the angle of back to hip is straight, rather than at forty-five degrees. I suggest that people straighten up their car seats as much as possible. There doesn't seem to be any solution to the discomfort of driving a car when you've got a pain in your legs except to get out and let somebody else drive! But you can sit straighter and relieve that discomfort now and then by walking around. The person who is humped over while writing or typing should stand up, bring the shoulders back and breathe deeply every hour. Otherwise he's going to be a humped over little old man if he doesn't remember to take care of his back.

I sometimes work with people who are using medication prescribed by their physicians. Some people will come to me and say, "Can I take this along with my valium?" I'll say, "How long have you been on valium? Are you experiencing side effects?" And I may give them something to counteract the side effects. Because valium is destructive to nerve tissues I give them supplements to heal the nerves. I'm conscientious about asking them if they're taking other drugs, and I may say, "You'll find out that you'll need a smaller dose. You won't be leaning on this so much. So be aware and see if you're doing better." I don't just say, "Quit taking the valium", because they often will gradually desire to quit on their own.

Sometimes people bring in vitamins for me to check out. Some of the vitamins on the market are not good because they're made from inorganic matter or are not readily assimilated. Take bone meal, for instance. The label says you can take bone meal to replenish the calcium in your body. But few people have good enough digestive juices to break down bone meal.

When selecting vitamins, people should look at the labels and find a brand made from a natural food source. If the calcium comes from milk, calcium lactate, or calcium carbonate then that's o.k.; that's from milk; that's a food; you can digest it. Some combinations of vitamins work well together. And there are different sources for the same vitamins as well. Vitamin A is found in cod liver oil, which is a fish liver oil. It also is found in carotene which comes from carrots. But in a great many cases oil is hard to digest. So if a person is under twenty-five I wonder, are they going to digest oil? I may not give them cod liver oil. I may give the vitamin A in dry tablet form not a capsule, and it won't tax the liver, but it will be digested. If I give cod liver oil, the liver may object. There may be an undesirable side effect. So I must know the patient well. If there's gall bladder distention and stones are forming, I must be careful. I don't give vitamin E oil either; I give it in dry powdered form.

## Vitamins

As a doctor, I am able to prescribe superior combinations of vitamins that can be fully used by the body tissues, along with some occasional aid from herbs. Russian radish is a fine herb. Outside it looks like a black carrot. Inside, it looks like a radish, whitish grey. It tastes peppery, like horse radish. The liver, the digestive tract and the stomach just love it. It stimulates all the digestive glands to empty out their enzymes. When it's used, very little thick bile forms, and no stones in the gall bladder. The bile doesn't stay in the gall bladder long enough to thicken. So I often give that little herb in tablet form.

Certain vitamins are best with food and others are not. It takes a bit of knowledge to know which. Calcium, for one, doesn't have to be taken with a meal. Vitamins A and E do have to be taken with a meal. Some can be taken on an empty stomach. Some herbs are taken only with water. For instance, if the kidney is clogged with uric acid crystals, you'd want to drink a full glass of water and take asparagus powder tablets in order to flush out the kidney; or a patient could cook asparagus and use some of the cooking juices for soup or tea; and serve some of the asparagus cold as a salad. I would have them do this three times a week.

I'm interested in arranging the diet to meet the needs of their physical health at that moment. It's fun to do and it involves the patients in doing something good for their bodies. If they like refreshing drinks, they can drink cranberry juice which aids the bladder. When they return for a visit to me they have taken care of themselves; they have taken my suggestions on vitamins; the metabolism is stimulated and their problems really improve.

No one is resistant to feeling better. But sometimes they're resistant to my diets! Some of the things they give up are status symbols like steak and baked potatoes. I want them to find restaurants that serve vegetables too. Not everybody likes Chinese food. But Mexican food contains a lot of vegetables, and so does chef's salad.

## Psychological Causes

There is a lot to the idea of psychological causes of physical ailments. At the menopause women enter a time of life where they take an assessment of themselves and their lives. Until that time they have cared very much about what people think of them. They want to look right in front of their families. They don't want to disappoint their parents. Their peers are very important. They want to make some progress and make some sort of a name for themselves. When they get to the menopause, they often become ready to chuck whatever people might think and lean on old age: "I'm old now. It doesn't matter. I can be as eccentric as I like." But there's a little adjustment period. There's a disappointment period. There's a depression. And it does have something to do with the body functions. The hormones are shifting gear, but the mind is involved, too. This body is one body, so I take the holistic approach. Some stimulus to the mind will help the adjustment. Turn your interest somewhere. Perhaps education. Perhaps art. Perhaps another family needs some help.

It's not only women in the menopause who have psychological and physical difficulties; it can be men or young people too. Do young people want to rebel against their parents and society forever, or do they want to take care of themselves? I try to show them that their parents just want them to be successful. I'm nobody special to them so I can say hard and harsh things and they may listen to me. I'm not a blood relative that has been lecturing them for years. I take this opportunity to tell them, and often it does work. Then I'll soften it a bit by telling them, "Look, I'm going to give you a nerve tonic, some $B_1$ or $B_6$; watch yourself. If you're full of anxiety, take some of this valerian. It is an herb with few side effects. Take this to ease your depression, to help you rest. Then make decisions." One of the biggest problems many people have today, even the President of the United States, is that they often can't make a decision before they go to bed. So all night long the wheels are turning. If they could simply make a decision just for today, and then make the next decision tomorrow, it might simply be an adjustment on today's decision and so it would go, day by day. If you can adjust your life so that you make only so many decisions today, and shelve the unimportant things, you have a happier nervous system. Don't leave things hanging. That can make you sick, give you ulcers.

## Transition

In certain cases I consider traditional allopathic medicine to be complementary to my work. I would not hesitate to call on an M.D. for an opinion and services in an applicable case. Certainly the first aid measures, the emergency room with its life sustaining equipment, broncho dialators, heart stimulants etc., are advantages I would not want to live without, nor without skilled surgeons to perform necessary operations. Allopathic medicine has developed pain killers which can be merciful to the human family. Pain, however, is a warning signal that indicated trouble somewhere in the body so I am cautious about the masking of symptoms that need to be treated with a corrective therapy.

The key factors in a healthy life are really quite simple. The person's psychological approach and their nutritional approach are the two key factors. We need to eat nourishing food and to maintain a happy outlook. A person who is agitated and anxious cannot digest food; if a person is full of anxiety about their job, their spouse, and their children, they'll be unhappy with themselves.

Or maybe they don't look the way they think they should. Maybe they eat their hearts away because they're a little heavier or a little skinnier than the conventional form and they're anxious. They sit down to eat but forget that we have only one liter of digestive juices in our bodies with which to digest food each day and that as we grow older our bodies make less juice so we must eat a little less. Anything you eat that exceeds the digestive potential of that one liter ferments and is not digested, which leads to problems. Health is a measure of the amount of nutrients the body assimilates and the joy of living the individual emanates.

**Exercise may often make the difference between leading an active, pain-free life and being contorted and disabled.**[18]

—Leon Root, M.D.; OH, MY ACHING BACK

# Exercises After Injury

This section of exercises is for people who have injured their backs and are interested in healing themselves through a gradual program of building strength and flexibility in their back muscles, and in the other parts of the body which support their backs. Among the more important things to think about when you're exercising after injury is to never strain yourself. Pace yourself. Move slowly and smoothly. It's especially important to breathe well as you do your movements, because proper breathing helps improve circulation, which in turn helps heal strained muscles and sore nerves. Breathing properly as you move also reduces emotional tension, which often heightens back problems. Remember to inhale as you stretch out and exhale as you curl in or contract. Also, while doing exercises lying on the floor, you may want to place a pillow under your pelvis so that the tendency to arch your back is reduced.

If you've had any kind of back injury, don't participate in violent or rigorous sports. And never do the Yoga exercises called the "plow" or the "shoulder stand" because those two exercises are hard on your back in every way. More people are injured doing them than doing any other exercises I know. As you exercise alternate spine arches in one direction with spine curls in the opposite. This alternating helps prevent strain or injury by balancing your muscle stretches. Whatever activity you're doing, always keep your knees slightly bent. Breathe fully. Try to reduce your anxiety and tension. Improve your diet. Take any kind of pain as a warning to lighten up, move more smoothly, and to do some simple corrective exercises.

You don't need to do many exercises at one time, or to do them fast. From doing even a few of them slowly each day, you'll see improvement.

## PHASE ONE OF HEALING

Phase one of healing is rest, until you feel no pain and your vitality appears to be returning. While resting you can stimulate your healing process by doing the breathing exercises and mental imagery described in the chapter in this book called Visualization. When you feel stronger try the exercises in this section.

The following is a series of simple exercises which anyone, no matter what kind of injuries they've had, should be able to do without harming themselves.

Be sure to do some gentle relaxation exercises first. You might do some meditation in order to relax before you begin the actual exercises, so that you release as much tension as you can before you begin moving.

## Isometrics

There are also several isometric exercises you can do where you simply contract and release your muscles without doing any kind of limb movement. These are beneficial after injury because they strengthen your muscles and improve your posture, without the risk of straining during movement.

Contract the muscles in your abdomen and your buttocks at the same time so that your pelvis tilts forward, and your stomach muscles share the job of supporting your spine and upper body. Contract and release these muscles with your breathing.

Lie on your stomach. Tighten your lower back muscles so that you can feel them contract from your tailbone up toward the top of your sacrum and waist. This contraction may make you arch your back slightly. Inhale as you contract and exhale as you release.

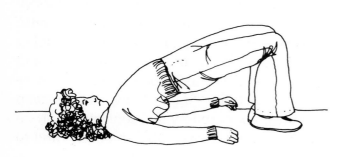

### The Pelvis Tilt

This is one of the most essential corrective exercises for low back problems and doing it can help improve or even eliminate lumbar lordosis. Lie flat on your back on the floor with your arms relaxed at your sides. Bend your knees and keep your feet flat on the floor. Then flatten your entire spine against the floor; raise your buttocks up off the floor by contracting the muscles of your abdomen and buttocks. Inhale as you lift your pelvis. Exhale as you let it come down again, making sure you lower your vertebrae at your upper back and waist first and then the others down to your tailbone.

This exercise helps to strengthen the gluteus maximus muscles in your buttocks, which help support your spine. It also helps prevent sway back, or lumbar spinal curve. If you have an occupation in which you must stand for long periods of time, doing this exercise will help you avoid back stress. If you are feeling weak you may want to do a less pronounced pelvic tilt than the one in the illustration. Work up to the full tilt gradually.

### Knee Lift

This helps limber the iliopsoas muscles. Lie on the floor with your arms relaxed at your sides or on your chest. And as you inhale, raise one knee toward your chest. Exhale as you bring your leg down again. Then repeat the movement with your other leg. When doing this be sure to keep your spine flat against the floor. Don't arch your back. Next, do this with both legs and re-member your breathing. You can hold onto your knees with the palms of your hands and draw your knees toward your chest and balance them there. This helps stretch out stiff muscles, ligaments, and joints in your lower back and is very relaxing.

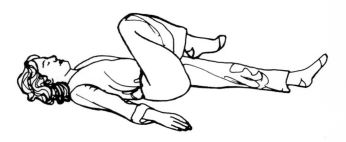

### Torso Stretch

This exercise is designed to stretch out the tight muscles on either side of your spine. Lie on your back, keeping your spine flat on the floor. Place your arms behind your head and rest your head on the palms of your hands. Bend your knees and keep your feet flat on the floor. Then cross your right leg over your left leg, using your right leg to draw your left leg down toward to your right. Draw both legs as far toward the floor as possible without straining. Bring your knees up again and uncross your legs. Reverse the process by crossing your left leg over your right and roll-ing both legs to the left. This limbers your hip joints and helps to open up your rib cage and stretch the muscles on either side of your spine.

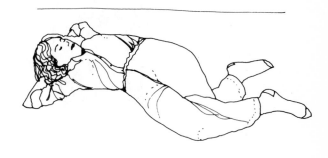

### Sacrum Roll

While you're in this position, with your feet flat on the floor, legs uncrossed and your knees together, roll your hips from side to side so that your knees move from left to right. Inhale as your knees come to the center in line with your spine. Exhale as your knees move to either side. You'll feel this opening up your middle and lower back.

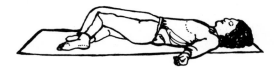

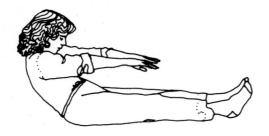

### Partial Sit Up

Lie down on the floor. Rest your palms on your chest. Inhale as you raise your head, neck and upper back off the floor, extending your palms toward your knees. Hold this outstretched position as you count to five. Then very slowly return to the starting position by lowering your back, then your neck, then your head, and finally your arms to the floor. Always keep knees slightly bent.

This exercise strengthens your abdominal muscles which are a major support for your lower back. It also strengthens your lower back muscles. It's a good exercise to do when you have had a back injury serious enough that full sit ups are not advisable.

### Torso Hang

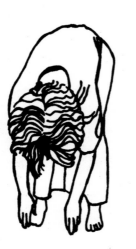

Stand up. Spread your feet about hip width apart. Relax your head and neck forward. Then slowly, vertebra by vertebra, curl your spine forward so that your arms are relaxed in front of you reaching toward the floor. Keep your knees slightly bent and try to touch the floor with your fingertips, but don't strain. Don't stretch, pull, or push your muscles. If you're not comfortable touching the floor, just approximate the position. You can allow your arms to swing gently while you hang to loosen your back as you breathe.

## PHASE TWO OF HEALING

The following exercises can be done when you're feeling stronger and you feel you can move on to slightly more vigorous exercise.

### Knee Kiss

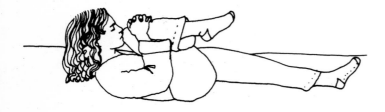

This exercise is a variation of the sit up. Lie on your back on the floor with both legs extended. Inhale as you bend one knee and draw it toward your chest, while you raise your upper back, your head and your neck off the floor. Now reach for your knee with your hands and draw it toward your face. From here you should be able to easily kiss your knee! Exhale as you release this position slowly until you are lying flat on your back again. Rest for a few seconds. Then try this movement with the other leg.

### Leg Scissors

This exercise helps strengthen muscles in your abdomen, hips and back. Lie on your back, keeping it flat against the floor. Put your head in the palms of your hands, and relax your elbows on the ground. Inhale as you raise both legs in the air. Then make a scissors motion with your legs, breathing in and out. Doing this for even a few seconds will help to strengthen your hip muscles and to release tension there. Do it with a pillow under your hips.

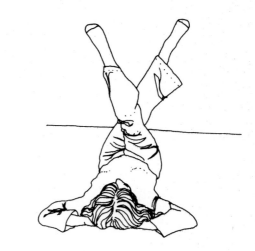

### Walking Backward

Another exercise for strengthening your hip, buttock and lower back muscles is done lying on your stomach with your head resting on your hands folded under your chin, or your head turned to one side, arms at your sides. As you inhale, raise one leg up behind you keeping the leg straight. Take care not to arch your back as you lift. Hold the leg about twelve inches from the floor for a count of ten. Then lower it to the ground as you exhale. Repeat with the other leg. Don't do this exercise until you are feeling very strong.

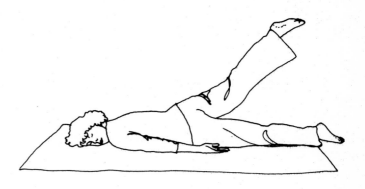

### Neck Lift

Because the neck is the upper spine, you can't separate neck pain from back problems. Neck pain is also often an early symptom of lower back problems. This exercise helps heal neck problems.

Lie down on your back on the floor. Flatten your spine; bend your knees, and keep your feet flat on the floor. Then place both hands behind your head. Bend your elbows and point them toward the ceiling. Use your hands and arms to lift your head off the floor, and curl your neck and head forward so that your chin is moving toward your chest. In this position, rotate your head to each side several times, keeping your chin as close to your chest as you can. Try to touch your shoulders with your chin. Stretching your neck and upper back this way will release deep neck tension; the stiffness and pain that you may feel will disappear if you do this exercise regularly.

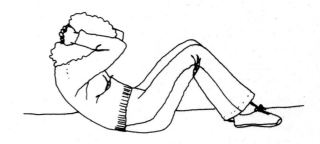

## Blade Squeeze

If you have injured or weak shoulder and upper back muscles, or spend long hours at a typewriter, a piano, or desk, this is a helpful exercise. Lie on your back on the floor. Clasp your hands behind your head, this time with your elbows flat against the floor. Then try to draw your shoulder blades together as you inhale and lift your chest slightly off the floor, arching your back. When you have squeezed your shoulder blades together as tightly as you can, hold them in that position for a few seconds. Now let your shoulder blades move outward again, flatten your back and release all your muscles as you exhale. Repeat the sequence several times.

## Arm Stretch

Lie on the floor on your back. Bend your knees, keeping your feet flat on the floor. Raise your right hand over your head and place your palm on the floor behind you. Stretch your extended arm behind your head as far as you can as you inhale. Then stretch the arm resting at your side toward your feet, so that your arms are stretching in opposite directions. Notice how this opens up muscles in your back that you don't often release. Hold that position for several seconds and then relax. Reverse the position and repeat the movement. This exercise improves the range of motion in your shoulders.

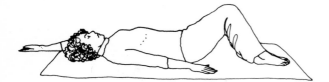

## The Standing Squat

Squatting keeps your knees, thighs, and other leg muscles strong, and keeps all the joints in your legs and hips limber, so that you can stand and lift using your leg muscles, rather than your back muscles. A variation of the floor squat is the "standing squat." Hold on to the edge of a counter, strong chair, or table that's waist height. Begin a movement cycle so that you inhale as you stand up and exhale as you squat down. Keep your back straight and your pelvis tucked under. Be sure not to arch your back. Keep your heels flat on the floor for as long as possible, while you're squatting down, only raising them when your hips get close to the floor. Then sit on the heels and rest in that position for a few seconds. Now inhale and stand up. This is also a good shoulder and upper back release.

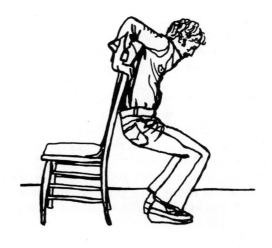

## Cervical Stretches

Next are exercises for removing stiffness in, and increasing circulation to the cervical and lumbar regions and the shoulder muscles. These exercises also stimulate circulation of the thyroid and parathyroid glands and relieve congestion and cramps in the shoulder muscles.

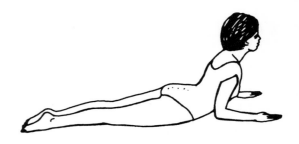

## The Small Cobra

Lie on your stomach on the floor. If you like, you can place a small pillow under your waist so that you back doesn't arch. Place your arms at your sides and lift your neck, head, and upper chest off the ground. Look up toward the ceiling as you raise your neck and your upper chest as high as you comfortably can. Hold that position for a few seconds. Relax your chest, then your neck, then your head down to the floor again. Depending on your condition, you can also do this exercise with your hands clasped behind you instead of on the floor.

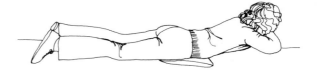

The exercise just described is a simplified version of the full Cobra, a Yoga asana in which you lift your whole torso off the ground barely using your arm muscles. You inhale as you arch and lift your torso, and exhale as you come back to the ground. But you shouldn't start attempting to do the full Cobra until your back has been strengthened by doing more limited arches.

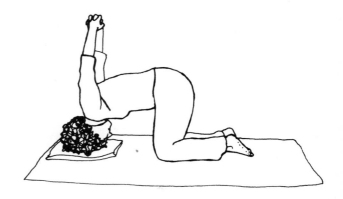

## Wing Back Stretch

Kneel and place a pillow about three feet in front of you. Clasp your arms behind you and rest them on your lower back. As you exhale, gradually lean forward to touch your forehead to the pillow while you bring your clasped arms up behind you, pointing them toward the ceiling. Reverse the motion and relax. This exercise helps open up your chest, helps relieve neck and upper back tension, and makes your shoulder muscles more flexible.

### The Shrug

Now stand up, place your feet shoulder width apart and do the "shrug." Inhale and raise your shoulders as high as you can toward your ears. Then exhale and push them behind and down, bringing your shoulder blades as closely together as you can. Then relax your shoulders as you return to your starting position. Don't thrust your head forward while you're doing this exercise. Keep it up and keep your neck as straight as you can. If you have pain or stiffness in your shoulders or neck do this exercise often to loosen them up. You can do it at work, in the car, or almost anywhere.

### Corrective Rests

If while doing your exercises, you feel any pain or stress, stop what you're doing immediately, take several deep breaths, and curl up into a fetal position on your side on the floor which is the least stressful position for your back.

Or if it feels comfortable, squat, and curl up with your arms between your knees, clasping your hands and resting your forehead on them. Then rock back and forth (not side to side) in this position as you breathe.

An excellent lower back release is to rest with the weight of your lower legs on a bench or chair.

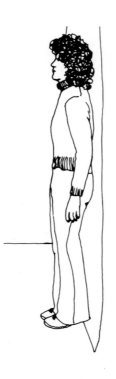

### The Wall Press

This standing exercise is a variation of other back flattening exercises done lying down. Place your buttocks, your heels, your shoulders and your head against a wall. Then press your whole spine, from your lower back to your neck, backward. See if you can flatten against the wall. Press as you exhale, then inhale when you've relaxed and released.

### Kneeling Ballet

When you're feeling slightly stronger a pleasant exercise is to get down on your hands and knees; as you inhale, lift one arm in front and the opposite leg behind, and look up. Exhale, come back down on your hands and knees, letting your head and neck relax down in front of you. Repeat the lifting motion with the opposite arm and leg. Make the movements smooth and continuous so that they become a kind of dance.

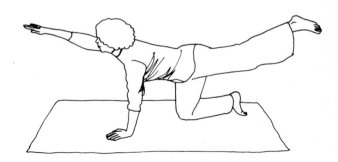

### Relaxation

In between exercises, often lie down on the floor and relax completely. Do this also throughout your exercising, so that you never strain yourself, you always keep within your limits, and you are refreshed rather than exhausted by what you're doing.

After you finish your exercises, lie on your back with your knees over your chest, your palms slipped between your calves and thigh muscles, holding your knees comfortably. Close your eyes. Let your breathing relax your torso and your stomach; relax all the muscles in your body, and experience the pleasure and benefit of the exercises you've done. Feel your whole body tingling slightly and feel the increased suppleness of your muscles.

## PHASE THREE OF HEALING

Here we begin a new section of more rigorous exercises to try once you have done the gentler exercises described comfortably for a while. When you feel that your back and the rest of your muscles are strong enough that you can go on to more rigorous exercises, incorporate the movements in this section in your routine.

### Cow-Cat

On your hands and knees, inhale as you look up at the ceiling, and let your middle and lower back sink down toward the floor, and arch your pelvis upward. (The cow.) As you exhale, curl your head and neck forward, tuck your pelvis under and arch your middle back up toward the ceiling, like a Halloween cat. Alternate these positions with your breathing. Make the movements smooth and continuous.

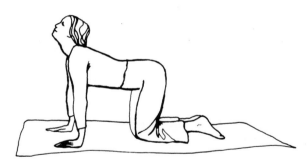

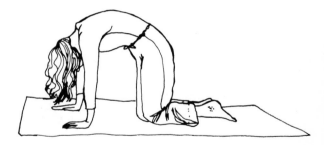

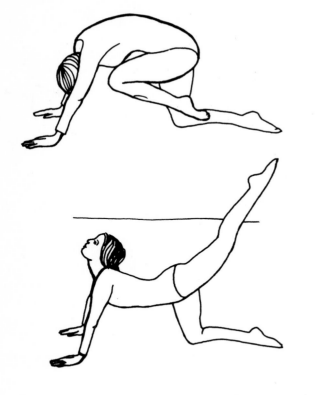

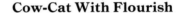

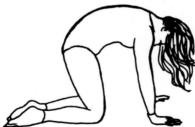

## Cow-Cat With Flourish

One exercise which incorporates balanced spinal movement is a variation of the yoga exercise, the "cow-cat." Beginning on your hands and knees, inhale and extend your right leg behind you. Now exhale as you bend your right knee and bring the knee toward your chest, curling your neck forward and bringing your nose as far toward your knee as you can. Then relax on your hands and knees. Now try the same sequence with the other leg.

## Andrea's Variation

My friend, Andrea, in Detroit showed me a variation of the cow-cat which she does to ward off low back problems. Kneel on your hands and knees with your head and neck relaxed forward and your pelvis tucked under. Alternate moving your pelvis from side to side (left to right), with making full circles with your pelvis in both directions.

## Jump Rope

Once you've become very strong, jumping rope is an excellent back exercise because it develops flexibility in your hip joints, your knees, and your lower back. It helps coordinate this flexibility with flexibility in your arms and shoulders. It's also good for your circulation. Remember to inhale as you raise your arms and exhale as you lower them.

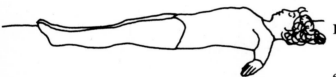

## Rest

Lie down and relax between all strenuous exercises.

## Swimming: The Panacea

Swimming, of course, is the best exercise that you can do for your back. My sister, an artist in New York, has managed to control a back problem by making sure she swims several times a week in an indoor pool. Her successful efforts convince me that beneficial exercise can be arranged even in the most hectic urban settings. The only caution about swimming is not to arch your back as you do the crawl, and to avoid doing the breast stroke until you're feeling really strong because it's hard on your lower back. Swimming teaches you to have very smooth movements. The water supports you; it takes a lot of strain off your body. If at all possible, swim every day. And try practicing some of these exercises in the water so that you can learn how they feel if you move really smoothly. See if you can recreate the smoothness of swimming movements when you do your exercises at home.

## Variety Is

Once you're feeling strong and healthy again, if you're the kind of person who prefers to have just one exercise so that you don't have to think about what you're doing, then do the Salute to the Sun exercise described in the Prevention section of this book. It is the most complete and effective exercise I've found. Be sure to do it slowly, smoothly and only a few times to start so you don't strain. Then increase your sequence to the full twelve times. If you get bored with one exercise, remember there are many, many exercises you can do. Pick any of the exercises in this book, or do them all for a short time, or change and focus on one or two of them a day. Remember not to stop exercising when you feel healthy and strong again. The process is responsible for much of your strength and vigor so keep it up! You'll continue to feel better and better.

\*　\*　\*

**It's never too late to start moving.**
　　　　　　　　　　—Meg M. Stern

\*　\*　\*

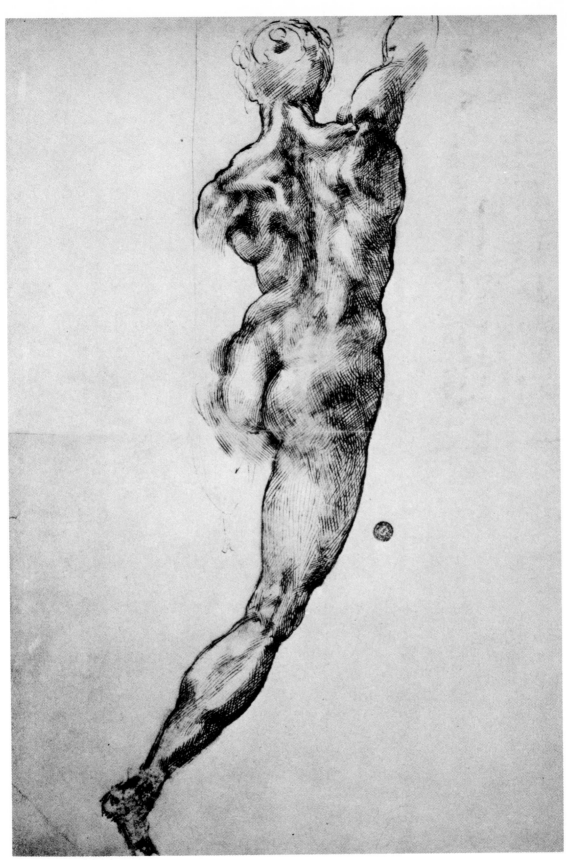

Study by Michelangelo

# VI
# Resources

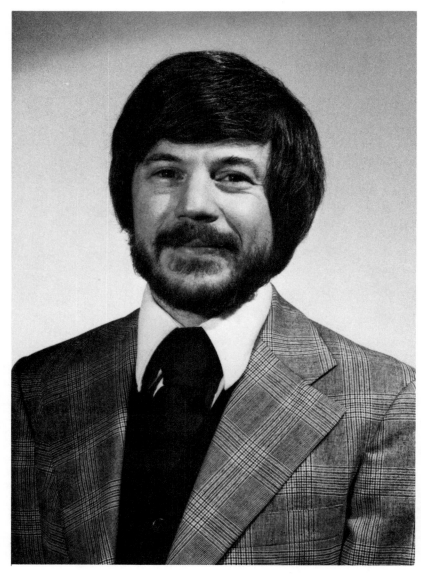

Richard Sindell

Vincent Buchanan

230

# A Personal Injury Lawyer: Richard Sindell

Richard Sindell is a graduate of Cornell University (1958) and Columbia Law School (1961). He has been in private practice since 1967 in Seattle, Washington. His practice is limited to the representation of people who suffer personal injuries resulting from medical and dental negligence; unsafe products, slips and falls and sports; automobile, pedestrian, motorcycle and other types of accidents caused by someone's carelessness. Sixty to seventy percent of his cases involve injuries to the neck or back. Most of the cases are settled. A small number go to trial. In addition to representing injured persons he has co-authored a chapter on paraprofessional handling of personal injury cases for the Washington State Trial Practice Manual, investigated disciplinary complaints against attorneys, and arbitrated fee disputes between clients and their attorneys for the Washington State Bar Association. He is on the roster of the American Arbitration Association to arbitrate uninsured motorist cases and is a member of the Association of the Trial Lawyers of America.

*Richard I. Sindell wishes to thank his uncle, Joe Sindell, an outstanding attorney who lives in Sebastopol, California, for his extensive assistance in writing this chapter.*

## Recovering Damages for Accidental Injuries

People suffer back and neck injuries at work, at home, in automobile accidents, by falling, in sports events and in other ways. The largest number of back and neck injuries occur at work and in automobile rear end collisions. If you are injured at work you have the right to recover a portion of your wage loss, and if you are permanently injured, you have the right to recover an amount of money determined by a schedule of benefits based upon the degree of your permanent disability. If you are injured on the job as a result of the negligence of someone other than a co-employee, or as a result of using a defective product, you have the right to present a claim for damages against the responsible person or manufacturing company. If the claim is rejected, you have the right to bring a lawsuit. You have the same right to sue if you are injured outside of a job setting. However, the fact that you have the right to make a claim or sue does not necessarily mean you will recover damages either through a settlement or a verdict in court. It will be your legal responsiblity to prove that the party who caused your injury was negligent or the product was defective.

## To Sue or Not to Sue

With very rare exceptions, if you are injured on the job, you cannot bring a lawsuit against your employer. An intentionally inflicted injury is such an exception in some states. One of the main purposes of Workers' Compensation laws is to avoid litigation and to provide funds, as quickly as possible, to permit a worker to receive medical treatment and living expenses. Each of the fifty states has a Workers' Compensation benefit system for persons injured on the job. The benefits vary from state to state. During the worker's period of recovery the formula for the payment is usually based upon wages earned at the time of the injury, but in some states all workers receive the same fixed sum regardless of their wages. There is also an award for permanent partial or total disability based on the percentage of the body disabled, as determined by a physician.

Although it is not necessary for you to establish that your employer or co-employee was negligent, there are three basic requirements you must satisfy to establish the right to participate in a state or insurance compensation fund:

1. The injury must be due to an accident.
2. The injury must be causally related to work being performed.
3. The injury must have occurred during the course and scope of the employment.

You can sue a third party, someone other than a co-employee, if that person negligently caused your injury. For example, if you are employed to deliver your employer's products or services, and you are involved in a vehicular accident, you can sue the negligent operator of the other vehicle, and the person's employer, if the other driver was acting within the scope of his employment. If you are injured because equipment is unsafe in design or defectively manufactured you can sue the manufacturer. For example, a punch press operator may suffer a severe hand injury because the press lacks a guard to keep his or her hands away from the punch.

In just two or three states an injured worker is permitted to keep both the state compensation and any funds obtained by way of settlement or verdict from the negligent third party. However, in other states, the state fund or insurance company who paid the Workers' Compensation is entitled to be reimbursed from the proceeds of any money received from the third party.

The reason for making a claim against the third party and suing, if necessary, is that your recovery of damages generally will be substantially greater than the scheduled Workers' Compensation benefits paid by the state or a private insurance company on behalf of the state.

If you are injured on the job, it is advisable for you to file a timely Workers' Compensation claim to insure prompt payment of all medical bills and replacement of a substantial portion of the wage loss. Each state, by law, limits the time for filing a claim to a year or some other period. Workers' Compensation payments are like a loan against the proceeds of a successful claim or lawsuit, but, in the absence of recovery from a third party, do not have to be paid back. Generally, at the conclusion of a case, the state or insurance carrier which has paid the Workers' Compensation claim will share in the payment of the attorney's fees and costs of the trial as well as receiving a part of the proceeds. Every large community has a group of lawyers which specializes in the handling of Workers' Compensation cases. The names of those particular lawyers can be obtained from the personal injury lawyer you retain to handle your case. If there is a third party claim to be filed, both the Workers' Compensation lawyer and your personal injury lawyer will be able to work together. Sometimes the same lawyer will handle both cases.

## Making a Claim; Employing a Lawyer

Your legal right to recover payment for injuries caused by another person's carelessness includes payment for the following elements of damage:

1. All out-of-pocket expenses, including medical treatment, hospital care, medicines, physical therapy, appliances and home care;

2. Income losses suffered from the time of the occurrences causing your injury to the date you returned to work;

3. Future income losses you are likely to suffer if your injury is permanent and has disabled you on a partial or permanent basis;

4. Payment for pain and suffering caused by the injury from the date it was incurred until

you recover, or if the injury is permanent, for your projected lifetime, which is computed by the use of standard life expectancy tables recognized by the courts. Pain and suffering includes the loss of enjoyment of life, which covers interference with recreational activities, sex and hobbies in additional to actual pain. It also includes any emotional problems which were caused, triggered, or aggravated by the injury producing event.

The one very important difference between a Workers' Compensation case and a third party claim or lawsuit is that you are entitled to recover an award for the pain and suffering that you experienced as a result of the injuries caused by the third party. A judge or jury determines the amount. In a Workers' Compensation case, the worker is paid a fixed sum of money according to a state statute which considers only the impairment of the ability to work and excludes compensation for pain and suffering.

It is most judicious for an injured person to retain a competent and experienced personal injury trial lawyer who will know how to evaluate injuries, tabulate the appropriate and collectible damages, and, if necessary, bring the case to trial. In addition to your own testimony about mental and physical pain, suffering and the ways in which the injuries have affected your ability to function and to enjoy life, damages must be established by proper proof through testimony by experts, including doctors, physical therapists, psychologists, economists, actuaries, and by friends, relatives and coworkers.

There is no law which prohibits you from representing yourself or handling your own case through to settlement or trial. It is, however, in this writer's opinion, the inappropriate thing to do. Expert knowledge is required on evidentiary and legal matters. The injured person should spend his or her time and effort recovering from the injuries and leave the matter of recovering damages to an attorney.

## Choosing Your Attorney

It is critical to the success of your case that you select a lawyer who specializes in handling personal injury matters. There are many ways for you to find the right lawyer. You may go to the courthouse in your community and ask the court bailiffs and clerks for the names of the lawyers who try lawsuits for injured people. Ask which lawyers they would select if they suffered personal injuries. Ask the trial judges the same questions. Usually they will give you a list of several attorneys' names. Your family lawyer and doctor are additional sources of information. You should make an appointment to see the attorney most recommended by the court personnel, your friends, neighbors, fellow workers, relatives, family doctor or lawyer or others.

Ask the attorney direct questions about his or her experience. What types of cases does s/he handle or specialize in? Does s/he try lawsuits? How often? How many? With what success?

Your choice of counsel should be based in large part upon your evaluation of the attorney as a person and his or her competence.

Determine if the attorney has compassion and understanding for injured people. Does s/he answer your questions directly and fully? Does the attorney appear interested in helping you solve your problems and not too busy to spend time on your case? Does s/he explain the applicable law so that you understand the favorable as well as the unfavorable statutes and appellate court decisions involved? Is the attorney knowledgeable about the medical aspects of your case? It should not take you long to pick up good or bad vibrations while you discuss your case. You will get what some lawyers refer to as a "gut reaction" as to whether you like the attorney you are talking to or not. If you do not like the attorney, then continue your search for a lawyer with whom you are comfortable.

The selection of a competent attorney to handle your case is a critical choice which ultimately will provide a satisfactory result, or produce an unpleasant experience and a poor financial outcome.

It's important to note that the successful handling of a personal injury case can be quite difficult and complicated. Personal injury cases require an experienced attorney, highly skilled and schooled in the art of law, and knowledgeable about medicine, science, engineering, and the trial of such cases. If you are injured and feel the need for an attorney, use the same care and caution in selecting a lawyer as you would a surgeon.

## The Costs Involved

You have the right to request an attorney to handle your case either on a percentage or an hourly basis. Since most people cannot afford to pay their attorneys a substantial hourly rate each month as the work is performed, they prefer to have the attorney take the case on a contingent fee basis, which means the attorney generally charges between twenty-five and thirty-three and a third percent of the award for handling a claim which can be settled without a lawsuit, and thirty-three and a half to forty percent of the final award for taking a case to trial. Unlike an hourly rate, which is payable monthly regardless of the outcome of the case, a contingent fee is paid only upon the successful conclusion of the case. A contingent fee contract permits a person of little or no income to retain a competent attorney to pursue his or her rights and obtain remedies s/he would otherwise be unable to afford.

Attorneys usually charge an additional fee to handle the appeal if a favorable jury verdict is appealed by the defendent. Some lawyers charge forty percent of the award or more in complicated cases (involving medical negligence or product liability) in which the expenses and amount of time required to prepare the case are enormous and the client cannot afford to pay the costs until and unless the case is successfully concluded. Most attorneys will require a client who can afford to do so to pay the expenses of litigation as they are incurred. You owe the costs whether the attorney settles or wins the case or loses, but, as mentioned above, if the contingent fee case is lost, you owe no attorney's fees.

## Difficult Cases To Win

Lawyers generally do not wish to handle cases against doctors or lawyers or complicated product liability litigation against manufacturers, which are often the nation's largest most powerful corporations. In most cities, only a small percentage of the attorneys are personal injury specialists, willing to handle cases against doctors, hospitals, other members of the healing professions and manufacturers. While there is an occasional general practitioner who is as competent to handle personal injury cases as a specialist, these lawyers are quite rare. It is extremely difficult for you to know or learn which general practitioner has the education, experience and skill to do an outstanding job in a personal injury case. The safest choice is to select a specialist. Even a specialist will often shy away from small cases or those in which liability (proof of fault) is difficult or appears impossible. In some cases, liability is clear, but proving the injury or damage may be difficult. Among the cases lawyers do not like are those in which the injury resulted from a slip and fall or a recreational activity, and those minor back or neck injuries which cannot be verified by x-ray or other objective tests. Juries tend to feel a person would not have fallen if he had been looking where he was walking. Juries will often believe that someone who engages in a potentially dangerous sport, such as skiing, or who drives a motorcycle, assumes a certain amount of risk and so are not sympathetic to this type of litigant. Cases which involve traumatic neurosis, that is, psychosomatic overlay of a minor physical injury, are also very difficult for even an expert personal injury lawyer to handle. Judges and juries do not always understand or relate to the type of injury that is emotional in nature and does not show up on an x-ray, leave a scar or anything tangible to see. A jury may even disregard the testimony of a psychiatrist or psychologist.

The cases lawyers favor are those in which the injury can be easily demonstrated by x-ray (fractures) or electroencephalogram (serious brain injuries) or obvious injuries like burns, scars, paralysis or amputation of arms or legs.

Often the person with a neck or back injury appears to be quite healthy although s/he may be suffering severe pain, and is seen as a complainer who makes a bad impression. Juries are reluctant to make substantial awards in these cases.

If a trial lawyer agrees to represent you, then you have the right to rely on that attorney to handle the case with a high degree of professional skill and thorough preparation, despite the potential problems. Trial lawyers are motivated to win in order to feed their own egos and to establish a winning reputation. Such attorneys will not generally shy away from difficult cases. In many instances the injured person cannot afford to pay the high cost of a trial. Even on a contingent fee basis a competent personal injury attorney will invest his or her time and effort and funds to protect and pursue your rights.

## Suing Doctors Or Hospitals

You can sue a doctor or hospital in the event that an injury or aggravation of a pre-existing condition results from a doctor's, nurse's or other hospital staff employee's negligence, carelessness, or incompetence. A doctor's negligence may be in the form of unnecessary surgery, abandonment, improper diagnosis, improper treatment or other surgical error. A nurse's mistakes may be in dispensing medication, dropping the patient, failing to put up side rails on a bed or inadequately monitoring and reporting changes in a patient's condition. Allergic reactions arising from the improper prescription of medications can also form the basis of a claim for damages. With increasing frequency, patients are also filing lawsuits against the manufacturers of medical devices and appliances which fail and cause injuries. For example, a catheter, or an intermedulary nail used to pin a fracture may break and cause complications.

Doctors and hospitals, however, do not guarantee that patients will recover. If a complication like a wound infection develops apart from any negligent acts or omissions by the hospital staff or doctors, the patient has no right to recover damages. The patient must prove that the nurse's or other hospital employee's or doctor's medical care fell below the standard of practice in that region of the nation. If it did, then it is considered "negligence." Even if physicians testify that there has been negligent conduct, if they do not also testify that it either aggravated a pre-existing condition or caused a new problem, the individual will not be entitled to receive damages. Generally this proof must be in the form of testimony by physicians, which is often difficult to obtain.

In a very few instances, if the negligence is clear, an injured person can recover without the testimony of an expert. In most instances, the patient cannot recover damages either in settlement or in the form of a jury verdict unless qualified experts in the same field as the negliggent

member of the healing arts can and will testify for the injured person in court. The expert must indicate what injury occurred, testify that the cause was due to the defendant's negligence and describe the extent of the permanent or temporary injury.

Since medical advancements are occurring at a rapid pace, the injured person cannot hold the hospital or doctor to knowledge of medical research, unless it was performed and the findings reported in the medical journals prior to the occurrence of the medical negligence. If a new and more effective medical procedure is first used following the patient's injury at the hands of a doctor or nurse, the newer technique cannot be mentioned at trial since it would be unfair to the doctor or hospital.

## When A Lawsuit Isn't Possible

Every state has a statute of limitations which limits the time for filing a lawsuit against a defendant. The statute of limitations is generally two or three years, although in California it is a single year following the event which caused the injury. In some states, if the negligent act causing the injury is not discovered before the time runs out to file a lawsuit, then additional time is permitted in which to do so. For example, if a person undergoes surgery and the doctor leaves a pair of surgical scissors or a sponge or some other object inside the abdomen, (which has happened frequently) then a lawsuit may be filed within the statutory period, or an additional year after the date the condition becomes known. In some cases, a condition or the negligence which caused it is not discovered for many years following the surgery, for example when a physician errs but either is unaware or fails to disclose it to the patient. In some states the statute of limitations is extended beyond the usual period for persons who are under the age of majority, at the time of the injury, or are in the military service, or for other reasons.

A trial specifically offers the injured person his or her "day in court" to prove the case in hopes of recovering an adequate award from the judge or jury. The success or failure of recovery varies with the type of case brought, as well as with the type of injuries sustained. Injured persons win substantially more than fifty percent of their cases with the exception of slip and fall cases, medical negligence and sports related injury claims. Because jurors tend to be protective toward doctors, it is difficult to succeed in a medical negligence case. An experienced attorney is best qualified to advise you as to whether you have a case, and whether you should drop it, settle it, or try it to a judge or jury.

## Preparing The Case: Your Roles

When an attorney takes on a case involving an auto accident or other injury the attorney will require that you sign a fee agreement. The attorney will obtain all available information relating to the accident, including the details of the event that caused the injury; names of witnesses; details of the injuries; a complete tabulation of all out-of-pocket expenses incurred; detailed employment history and a medical history including prior injuries, diseases, and hospitalizations; and miscellaneous historical data including crimes committed by the client, if any.

The attorney will hire an investigator to talk to witnesses, obtain the police report, talk to the police officers and perform any other necessary investigation. The attorney will hire a professional photographer to photograph you in the hospital, your visible injuries, if any, and if permitted, the other driver's vehicle. The attorney will hire accident reconstruction, medical, and other experts if necessary, and if it would be helpful, refer you to orthopedic surgeons, internists, neurologists, psychiatrists, psychologists, plastic surgeons, or other medical specialists. The attorney will confer in person or telephone with you on a regular basis to obtain information regarding your medical progress, additional wage losses, subsequent accidents or diseases, and other valuable and necessary details. Do not wait for your attorney to inquire about these changes, however; contact the lawyer or a member of his or her staff and communicate the new information as soon as you acquire it. Your cooperation will make it possible for your attorney to follow your medical progress carefully. It will also enable him to make recommendations to assure that you receive the best possible medical care.

You must cooperate with your attorney in other ways; for example, in giving all the information he or she seeks. You must obtain the necessary medical treatment by staying in close touch with your doctor and following his or her instructions, the doctor's order to return to work in particular, even if you disagree, but cannot persuade the doctor. If, upon returning to work, you cannot function because of the pain, you can return to the doctor and tell him his or her order was premature.

One of the most important facets of the client-attorney relationship is frequent communication between client and attorney. The client must provide the attorney with the eyewitnesses' names, addresses and telephone numbers, and similar information regarding witnesses to the injured person's condition preceding and following the injury. The client must disclose all the essential and sometimes personal details of his or her life to the attorney so that all possible gaps in the preparation and presentation of the case can be bridged. Many a case has gone down to defeat because the client kept vital information from the attorney. Because the attorney-client relationship prohibits the attorney from revealing anything told to him by the client without the client's permission, the client is fully protected. No similar protection is possible when the defense lawyer cross examines the client unless the client's attorney is forewarned and can make the proper objections at the appropriate times.

As well as having the responsibility to give your lawyer information you have the right to receive information from him or her. It is best to retain an attorney who is not so busy that he or she will ignore your case. You should then trust the attorney's judgment. The attorney should give you progress reports so that you can feel assured there is progress. You can expect fair treatment at the hands of the attorney. You have the right to be kept fully informed of progress of your case and to receive photocopies of all relevant documents which the attorney prepares, or receives from opposing counsel. You have the right to inquire about your case at any time, within reasonable bounds, and to receive a prompt, detailed reply either from the attorney or the attorney's staff. If you do not receive this type of courteous, responsive service, you have the right to dismiss the attorney and retain another one. In extreme cases, you can and should complain to the local Bar Association in the event the attorney ignores you or your requests. Of course you as a client should not make unreasonable demands of your attorney, for he or she also has the right to dismiss you as a client.

Initially you should carefully interview the lawyer you select, should obtain a written fee agreement which you understand and have had the lawyer or his paraprofessional or secretary explain in detail, and should understand what you may expect in the form of communications to and from the attorney and his or her staff.

At the outset, you have the right to know whether the attorney will be handling the case personally or plans to turn it over to a younger associate. You have the right to refuse to have the attorney delegate the case.

You should participate in your case by attending as many meetings with experts, depositions, court hearings, and settlement conferences with insurance adjusters and opposing attorneys as possible. The purpose of this is to educate you to become an effective witness. You are also likely to appreciate knowing precisely what is happening in your case.

As soon as you have fully recovered and your doctor dismisses you, or your condition has stabilized, and the physicians are able to predict the future medical progress, you must inform your attorney, who may then attempt to settle your claim. If settlement is not possible, then counsel can file a lawsuit and proceed to prepare for the eventual trial.

If a claim can be settled without a lawsuit, the expenses you will ultimately be responsible for are substantially less and a settlement may occur years sooner than the case could be brought to trial. Many cases are settled in between the commencement of the lawsuit and the trial. Over ninety percent of all cases filed are settled without the need to go through a complete trial to verdict.

## Sports Injuries And Lawsuits

If you are an athlete you generally cannot sue your own team if you suffer an injury while engaged in the sport. However, it is quite possible that you may have a product liability claim against the manufacturer of a helmet or other sports equipment. If it can be shown that the equipment was unsafe and caused or contributed to an injury, there may be a chance to recover from the manufacturer or distributor. Most teams have insurance to cover the medical costs resulting from treatment for sports related injuries, regardless of the right to recover for pain and suffering and lost earnings from a third party.

## Accidents In The Home

You can definitely sue the manufacturer if a product used in the home was defective and caused an injury. In such a case you will be required to prove the product was defective and that that defective condition was the proximate cause of your injury.

Some states have comparative negligence statutes which will permit you to recover a portion of your damages, even though you are partially at fault. Other states allow you to recover as little as ten percent of your damages if you are judged to have been ninety percent at fault. Still other states will bar your claim if you are more than fifty percent responsible for your own injury. Generally the percentage of contributory or comparative negligence is determined when your case is negotiated with an insurance company or an attorney. In the event of a trial the jury will decide whether the product was defective, and in other types of injury cases, the issues of negligence and contributory negligence. If neither party requests a jury then the case can be tried by a judge. Judges are more likely to award damages, but the awards are generally more moderate than a jury of twelve of your peers is likely to give. Jurors can go to either extreme and award either substantially more or substantially less than a judge; they are more unpredictable. Your attorney will discuss the pros and cons of a jury or nonjury trial with you. In some cases it is best to let the jury make the determination and in others it is wiser to have the judge do so.

## Medicine's Participation

While there are many cooperative doctors, there remains a hard core of physicians who are too busy treating their patients to become involved in time consuming personal injury litigation. In Seattle, Washington, for example, a number of orthopedic surgeons will accept a referral from another doctor but will not assist an attorney unless their own patients are injured. They have no choice but to testify for their own patients; they can be subpoenaed. If an injured person starts with a general practitioner, that doctor can refer the patient to a specialist, including an orthopedic surgeon, a neurologist, a neurosurgeon, an internist or a doctor who specializes in physical medicine and rehabilitation (a physiatrist).

The difficulty in finding a doctor who is willing to testify at depositions and at trial is another reason for contacting a personal injury lawyer as soon after your injury as possible to do so. The lawyer you select should know the doctors in the community who specialize in the treatment of injured people and which doctors are willing to assist the patient's cause by way of deposition or trial. The American Medical Association has a set of rules concerning the duty owed by a doctor to a patient when that patient suffers injuries as a result of an accident. The rule is that the doctor is to cooperate with the patient's attorney, since it is part of the doctor's duty to attend to all of the patient's needs, including the lawyer's request for assistance, reports and testimony. The rule unfortunately is sometimes honored more in its breach than in its observance.

## Arbitration

It is a mistake to sign a form that waives your right to sue and forces you to arbitrate any claim which may arise as the result of negligence by nurses or other members of the hospital staff, and the doctors who treat you at the hospital. While arbitration is a less expensive form of obtaining an award, the awards are often inadequate. The arbitration panel generally consists of doctors and one or two lawyers. One of the lawyers is usually a defense attorney who represents doctors and hospitals for an insurance company. Usually the deck is stacked against the individual patient. The doctors who serve on the panel generally believe that every settlement or award against a doctor or hospital increases their own malpractice insurance premiums. They are quite naturally defensive about such claims. It is difficult to find objective doctors. There are some arbitration panels which are set up in a more balanced manner with fewer doctors and more attorneys. This type of panel is rare.

To sign an arbitration form waiving your right to sue is a very risky decision. It may be that at some time in the future arbitration panels will be the most desirable form of obtaining a just award but that is not yet the case. Although arbitration is more rapid and can be less expensive than a court trial, where there has been a serious injury, arbitration is not the desirable forum, although arbitration may be the best format for obtaining an adequate award in a small or medium size claim. There is no way for a patient who enters the hospital to know in advance what carelessness and injuries may occur in the hospital and, therefore, it is best not to waive the right to sue in favor of the right to arbitrate.

## Reasonable Expectations

You should be extremely cautious about retaining an attorney who makes great promises to obtain a specific dollar amount for you in a short period of time. Notwithstanding the fact that the Supreme Court of the United States is now permitting lawyers to advertise, be wary of lawyers who advertise that they obtain rapid settlements or obtain large verdicts, without first establishing that they are qualified to handle serious or even minimum value personal injury cases.

Cases vary so greatly that it is best not to have expectations concerning the outcome of your case; the amount to be received in settlement or awarded by a jury; the form of compensation, whether a lump sum or an annuity; or the time it will take to complete the handling of the claim or bring the case to trial. None of these matters can be determined until the extent of the injuries becomes clear and the damages can be computed.

A serious injury will require a far longer period for the injured party to recover or if complete recovery is not possible, for the medical condition to at least stabilize so that it can be evaluated by the doctor. It is best for the attorney not to bring a case involving a serious injury to a conclusion until either a medical determination that complete recovery has taken place is made or that the injury is permanent and disabling has been determined. A settlement or a jury award is final and you have no right to reopen the case. As a result, the highly competent attorney will not wish to bring a case to too rapid a conclusion for fear you will not receive an adequate settlement or award or be protected in terms of future damages.

In larger communities it takes between two and three years, and sometimes longer for a case to come to trial. Settlements can be obtained at any point during the waiting period. Despite your wish for a timely resolution of your claim, it is better to have a highly skilled attorney who will take longer to bring your case to trial than an incompetent one who will obtain a poor result in a shorter period of time.

## Difficult Cases

There are numerous ways in which a personal injury case can become difficult to win or situations in which an adequate settlement or jury verdict is unlikely. If there are no independent witnesses but you and the defendant, the case is likely to result in a standoff, with the defendant winning. The jury may not be able to decide whom to believe; since you as the plaintiff have the burden of proof, the defendant wins if the jurors reach an impasse. If you wait several years before going to an attorney, it is difficult to reconstruct the incident and prove damages.

There are those cases in which the injured person has gone to a general medical practitioner who does not honor his duty to his patient to testify at deposition or in court or to prepare a detailed medical report for the attorney handling the case.

There are cases complicated in terms of fault, which involve only minor injuries which are nondisabling and have no permanent effect upon the body or mind. This type of case is expensive to prepare for trial and has only a small potential recovery in damages.

If the injured person is a difficult individual who is likely to make a poor impression on jurors and refuses to follow the advice of the trial attorney to settle or to testify humbly, the result may not be a happy one for the plaintiff.

An easier case is one in which you are a pleasant, likeable person and have suffered an injury which is visible (a scar or other deformity) or have sustained a large provable loss of money for wages, medical bills and other damages. Jurors will want to give you a generous award. Other easier cases are those where the injuries are serious, suffering severe, fault is clearly that of the defendant and the insurance limits are sufficiently high to cover the damages.

## Common Misconceptions

Many of us have heard stories about people recovering huge sums of money for back and neck, and other types of injuries. Most of these stories are exaggerated. The fact that a newspaper article reports that a verdict of $100,000 was returned for someone who suffered a back injury does not mean that your back injury is worth a like amount. Every case is as unique as the person who is injured. Although the public is becoming better informed and more conscious of its rights, most people know very little about the medical-legal ramifications of personal injury claims and trials. All too often, the public is misled by what it sees on television or reads in the newspapers. Neither medium gives an accurate picture. In real life, Perry Mason would never win all of his cases in sixty minutes and in addition sell soaps, aspirin and hairspray every fifteen minutes.

Many persons also have misconceptions concerning their ability to represent themselves without the assistance of an attorney. The average person is no match for a well trained insurance adjuster. The unrepresented claimant is likely to obtain either no settlement or a grossly inadequate one. It is a mistake to represent yourself in any legal situation involving a claim for damages resulting from personal injuries. This saying, attributed to Abraham Lincoln, "The person who acts as his [or her] own lawyer has a fool for a client," still holds true. The insurance industry is in business to make a profit. They retain well trained adjusters and highly competent defense lawyers. Since you do not have to pay an attorney unless he or she succeeds in obtaining a result for you, what have you got to lose? Retain a lawyer and let him or her do your work on a contingent fee basis. Good Luck!

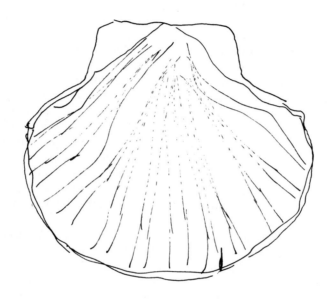

Water doesn't recognize any one spot as prettier or sexier than any other. Water wants it all.

—Lea Perrin, WET Magazine

# Spas and Hotsprings

\* \* \*

**Give me the luxuries and I'll dispense with the necessities.**
—Oscar Wilde

\* \* \*

This is an eclectic listing of some of the world's spas. As rates vary greatly, we recommend that you write for brochures and full information before making your reservation. You may also wish to investigate health clubs in your area. And, of course, there's always the good old Y (M or W) CA, where you may find pools, exercise classes, weight rooms, racquet ball and squash courts available to you for a reasonable membership fee.

The staff and facilities vary from year to year in the hospitals as well as the spas. These listings are not necessarily recommendations. Investigate each center for your own needs.

\* \* \*

Town of Bath, England
Roman baths (since 43 A.D.)
For information, write:
Tourist Information Centre
8 Abbey Churchyard
Bath, England

Merida Private Steam Baths
Merida is a city on the Yucatan Peninsula. The baths are in a hotel in the center of town. Massage, showers, steam rooms, swimming pool.

Village East Russian Baths
268 East 10th Street
New York, New York
Massage, swimming pool, Russian Steam Baths up to 250°, fresh spring water, cold showers. The Russian baths and the Russian food bar are the highlights. Delicious fresh melon and strawberries, creamed herring, smoked fish, pumpernickel, poppy seed cakes. Wednesday is ladies' day.

The Sanctuary
Covent Garden Tube Stop
London, England
Wood decor, luxurious, atmosphere. Solarium with sun lamps and sauna. Swimming pool with high ceiling, skylight, mirrored walls, perfumed water, black and white checked tiles, and a swing over the pool for dangling your toes. A highlight is what a friend calls "the MGM Room": small walkways cross over the 85° pool, surrounded by exotic flora and live splendid

parrots on perches; couches to lie on and feel like Jane Russell. Also a food and juice bar. In a good shopping area.

Margaret Island Thermal Spa
Budapest, Hungary
Spa in parks and gardens on an island just outside center of Budapest; swimming, dancing, tennis, yachting, thermal baths, gym, massage, restaurant, nightclub.

Thermal Hotel Heviz
Heviz, Hungary
Luxurious country spa; natural hot lake Heviz; medical exams, fitness programs, gyms, sauna, mud baths, massage; Hungarian cuisine.

Baden, Baden
Germany
A renowned health spa.

Town of Calistoga, California
Boasts six spas. All offering mud baths, hot mineral waters, sulfur steam and blanket wraps.

Campbell Hot Springs
Sierraville, California
Small concrete hot pools, indoor tubs.

Carson Hot Springs
1525 N. Ormsby Blvd.
Carson City, Nevada
98° mineral-water swimming pool, private baths, massage.

Arita Hot Baths
Wakayama prefecture, Japan
Unusual gourmet bathing: after shower, step inside a cable car on a high rocky cliff. The car contains eight small tubs of very hot water. As the car slips away from the cliff's edge, you soak in your tub and enjoy the view of surf far below. The cable car ride is about fifteen minutes of bath suspension before return.

The Golden Door
P.O. Box 1567
Escondido, California
Weigh-ins, walking, aerobic and pool exercises, gymnasium, sauna, Scotch baths, massage, dance/calisthenics classes, Yoga, herbal wraps, tennis, swimming, steambath, Jacuzzi, hot tubs, Tai Chi, vegetarian cuisine.

The Greenbrier
White Sulphur Springs, West Virginia
Golf, tennis, riding, swimming, bowling, trap and skeet shooting, mineral baths, massages, Scotch sprays, whirlpool and steam baths. Special "health" weekend: lectures on preventive medicine and low-cal cuisine; gorgeous West Virginia landscape.

The Greenhouse
P.O. Box 1144, Arlington, Texas
Indoor and outdoor pools, swimming and tennis lessons, facials, massage, sauna, whirlpool, individual exercise plans, manicure, pedicure, hair style and cosmetic consultation, low-calorie diet.

Grover Hot Springs
Near Markleeville, California
Two swimming pools 80°, 102°.

The Homestead
Hot Springs, Virginia
Golf, tennis, fly-fishing, skeet shooting, horseback riding, bowling, swimming, skiing, ice-skating, mineral bath, saunas, steam room, massage, whirlpool bath, Zander-gymnasium, exercise tank, sun lamps, hot packs, medical supervision.

Kabuki Hot Springs
Japan Center—Geary Street
San Francisco, California
Expert shiatsu massages and hot baths.

Maine Chance
Phoenix, Arizona
Paraffin wax bath, depilatory waxing, steam cabinet, sauna, whirlpool, body massage, exercise classes, pool exercise, cycle exerciser, rollers, vibrators, 900-calorie diet for weight loss, facials.

Orr Hot Springs
Orr Springs Rd., Ukiah, California
Hot spring filled tubs, cold water swimming pool.

Palm-aire Spa
Palm-aire Drive North
Pompano Beach, Florida
Hotel accomodations. Loofah scrub, Scotch spray, salt-glo rub, whirlpool baths, warm and cold contrast pools, herbal wraps, saunas, steam cabinets, Turkish bath, Swiss shower, Gymnasium, indoor and outdoor massage, Roman Bath, exercise pool, tennis, golf, solaria for nude sunbathing, medical exam by resident M.D.

Rancho La Puerta
Tecate, California
Massage, facials, herbal wraps, exercise, body awareness, spot reducing, stretch and posture work, Yoga, fitness classes, circuit training, water exercise, sauna, hot tub, lacto-ovo, calorie-controlled organic vegetarian cuisine, 3 meals a day.

River Inn
3400 W. 4th Street, Reno, Nevada
Combination motel, casino, bar and hot springs spa, outdoor and indoor pools @ 100°, steam room, Jacuzzi, private pools, and massage.

Safety Harbor Spa
Safety Harbor, Florida
Medical exam on arrival, individual diet programs, exercise classes, Yoga, gymnasium, whirlpool baths, physiotherapy, indoor mineral water pool, massage, mineral baths, solaria, Swiss and Danish showers, tennis, golf, bicycling.

Steamboat Hot Springs
16020 S. Virginia Street
(10 miles south of Reno)
Nevada
Mineral baths, steam room, blanket wrap, mud-pack and pool, massage and reflexology.

Tassajara Mountain Center
A Zen monastery in the Carmel mountains which allows visitors during the summer months, this is one version of earthly paradise. With lovely natural hot springs, steam saunas, delicious food, Japanese style cabins, meditation available, enchanted woods, friendly personnel and a waterfall-fed swimming gorge, one is tempted to convert!

THERMAL SPRINGS OF THE UNITED STATES & OTHER COUNTRIES: A SUMMARY

Geological Survey Professional Paper #492;
Available from:
Branch of Distribution, USGS
1200 South Eads Street
Arlington, Virginia 22202
$3.45
This book could be your ticket to the sybaritic pleasures of bathing in undeveloped hotsprings, of camping with hot (and sometimes cold) running water. Picture yourself unwinding in a geyser-fed pond with all creation unfurled before you, wild geese honking in the distance . . . Sound pleasant? Thank your friendly federal government for the directions.

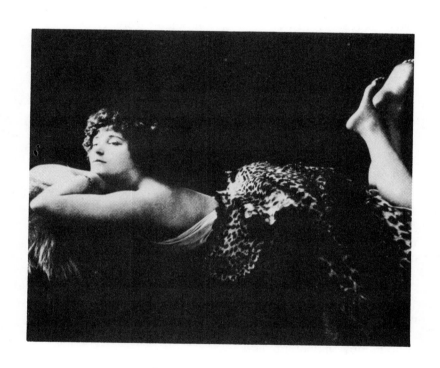

# Beauty and the Back

**You can see by the way people look if what they do is good for them.**

—Marion Rosen

From the excellent exercises you are now doing, your back is becoming more shapely and beginning to glow from improved circulation. You may want to enhance your health and enjoyment with massages, saunas, creams and herbs.

## Skin Deep

Take care to protect the skin of your back from too much sun on the beach or by the pool by using a strong sunscreen.

You can also protect your skin from harsh chlorine in pool water by applying the cream made by the recipe which follows. Dr. Evon Karanoff, who devised it, says it's "the most fantastic swimming cream known to us on the physical plane!" You can add Paba to it if you want. Apply it to coat your skin before swimming to prevent oil and vitamin loss.

## Massage Oil

You can make fine massage oil by combining one part almond oil and four parts unprocessed vegetable oil (from a grocery or health food store) with several drops of fragrant oil to your taste. Or you may prefer body powders as a massage lubricant.

## Swim Cream

1        jar anhydrous lanolin
4-6      bars of cocoa butter
oil of almonds as needed
rose water in proportion
2 oz.     glycerin

Melt cocoa butter slowly; put in blender with lanolin. Add glycerin and blend. Next add almond oil and rose water, in proportion to make the cream as heavy or light as you want. Pour into a jar and let it cool.

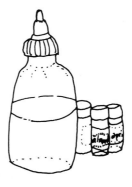

### In the Sauna

In a steamy Finnish sauna, apply a mixture of buttermilk and sea salt to a hot wash rag, and scrub your back. The salt cleans the pores and the milk supplies ingredients beneficial to your skin. Yogurt and almond meal mixed make a slightly less abrasive cleanser. Be sure to include your upper arms and the back of your neck in your scrub. Rinse with cool water to close your pores again.

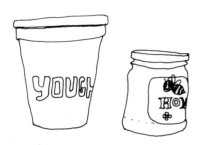

### Milk and Honey

The ancient skin panaceas of milk and honey are still unbeatable treats. You can apply yogurt or honey directly to your skin. Leave either of them on awhile so they can be absorbed. Then rinse with warm water.

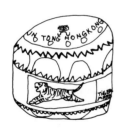

### Tiger Balm

Try Tiger Balm, a tingling, aromatic Chinese ointment that comes in beautiful jars. Apply sparingly to tense muscles. An ancient antidote for lack of energy is to scratch tiger balm into your skin along your ribs and back with a piece of jade.

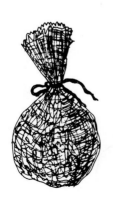

### Back Ache Shower

In her book, KITCHEN COSMETICS (Panjandrum/Aris Books), Jeanne Rose describes an herbal treatment for low back ache.

Use only dried herbs and mix them together. Combine large handfuls of these herbs in a muslin bag: rosemary leaves, sage leaves, strawberry leaves, comfrey root, comfrey leaves, and lavender buds. Close the bag. Soak the full herb bag thoroughly in water. Let a warm shower gradually get hot. Rub the herb filled sack on your skin from your feet up to your lower back with a circular motion. As you rub, alternate the water temperature on your lower back from one minute of hot spray to twenty seconds of cold spray. End the shower with a quick cold rinse, wiping your skin with the herbs.

\*    \*    \*

**In one part of Africa . . . the nails are coloured yellow or purple. In many places the hair is dyed of various tints. In different countries the teeth are stained black, red, blue, etc., and in the Malay Archipelago it is thought shameful to have white teeth "like those of a dog" . . . It is certainly not true that there is in the mind of man any universal standard of beauty with respect to the human body.**

—Charles Darwin, THE DESCENT OF MAN, 1871

\*    \*    \*

## Oils

Pure cocoa butter makes one of the best skin oils available. Massage your back and hips with it to help prevent wrinkles and soften your skin. Almond oil also softens the skin and is a fragrant pleasure.

## Clothes On Your Back

Be sure not to wear clothing which will cause your back to tense up. Besides being uncomfortable, a tense back is less beautiful. Choose clothes with loose waists so that your diaphragm muscles are not constricted. Girdles and clothes which fit tightly around your pelvis ruin the circulation in your hips and lower back, causing broken veins and stretch marks. Wear low-healed shoes, round-toed, wide enough not to pinch your feet. High heels and tight shoes throw your spinal alignment off and can cause lower and upper back pain. Flat shoes with good arch support are usually best for most feet.

## Backlighting

For more outrageous social moods try commercial skin creams that sparkle. Halston makes a beautiful skin sparkle in several tones that comes in a raindrop shaped jar. Dazzle them coming and going!

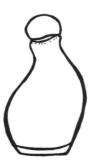

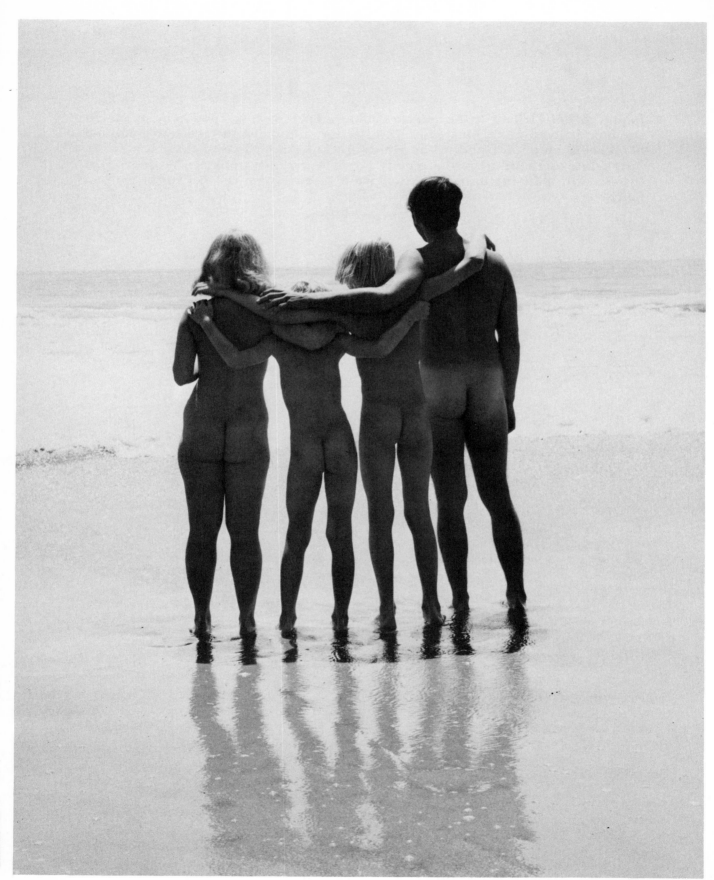

Elisa Bowen

248

# SOME BACK GEAR

### Pal-Relax-Bar

Pal-Relax Bar Co., 233 Oak Knoll Rd., Ukiah, California 95482. The bar is said to be useful in therapy of back pain and tension headaches. It's an exercise bar for your home. Large enough and strong enough to hang upside down from and do exercises. Many converts claim hanging inverted from the hips relieves spinal nerve pressure and realigns the vertebrae. Smaller exercise bars are available at department and sports stores.

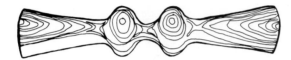

### Ma Roller

A wooden healing tool invented by an acupuncturist, designed to stretch the spine and massage surrounding muscles. You roll it over a muscle or lie down on it for massage. Great Earth Healing, Inc., 660 Elm Street, Montpelier, Vermont 05602; or Great Earth Healing, Ltd., P.O. Box 24, London SW115QF, England.

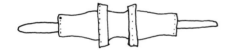

### Captain Carrot Caresser

Built on the same principles as the Ma Roller but better, I think, because it has foam rubber padding to cushion the wood's contact with your body. Bath Ma and the Captain are similar to plain old rolling pins which also feel good rolled on your muscles. Captain Carrot Caresser, P.O. Box 26999, Sacramento, California 95826.

### Japanese Spine Tapper

Called a pon-pon, it's a rubber ball on the end of a supple metal stick. Tap yourself or a friend on the back. As the ball bounces, your circulation and energy improve.

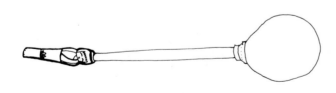

### Back Balls

Buy pretty colored rubber balls in small sizes (about 4″ in diameter) in a dime or toy store. Use them under your neck and to lie and sit on to relax muscles. (See Visualization chapter for exercise instructions.)

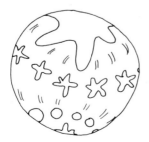

250

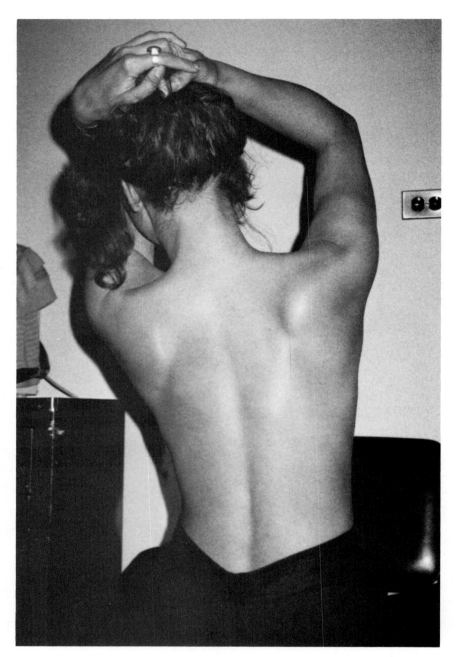

Evon Karahoff

# Back Matter

backlog
backbone
backsail
back row
backdrop
back down
backbite
backslide
moneyback guarantee
greenback
backarat
backgammon
backalaureate
back to school
backteria
backsword
backhand
backgate parole
kickback
backslap
backtalk
backless
backwoods
backwater
back alley
backdoor man
halfback
back cover
halfback
fatback
quarterback
knife in the back
fullback
backward personality
back number
back and fill
fastback
razorback
flat on your back
hunchback
humpback
swayback
back cross
backwardation
backwardization
double back
look back
feedback
double yr. moneyback

back off
backlet
backbond
backtack
backrest
backyard
back to nature
back in style
backdive
backswim
backspin
backstroke
Back Bay
backwash
backstep
outback
flashback
water offa ducksback
backhouse
backstrap
backfall
backstitch
backermost
backermore
backstay
back lot
back bar
Zwieback
backless
backlist
backboard
backalao
horseback
greenback
hardback
back matter
backformation
back court
back out
backlash
backside
backwoods
back page
back in the saddle again
back way
back and blue
back court
back to the wall
setback

backboard
backstairs
backhand
Backminster Fuller
backstretch
backlet
back to work
backtrack
backscatter
Back River
backseat driver
backstress
backsight
backcloth
backlight
paperback
wetback
backstage
backboard
backasswards
backswept
backstream
back atcha
backstage
backpack
back up
J.S. Back
comeback
playback
backfire
backfield
backbench
backanal
backlash
back door

# Back Clinics and Hospitals

Columbia University Hospital
New York, New York
Multiphasic back treatment services.

Industrial Injury Clinic
Theda Clark Memorial Hospital
Neenah, Wisconsin
Good rehabilitation center for back problems.

Orthopedic Hospital
Edinburgh, Scotland
Multiphasic back treatment services.

Pain Center Rush-Presbyterian—
St. Luke's Medical Center
Chicago, Illinois

Pain Management Center (Inpatient unit)
Mayo Clinic—St. Mary's Hospital of Rochester
Rochester, Minnesota

Chronic Pain Clinic (Outpatient unit)
Mayo Clinic
Rochester, Minnesota

Pain Center
Mt. Zion Hospital and Medical Center
1600 Divisadero St.
San Francisco, California

Pain Clinic
University of Washington
School of Medicine
Seattle, Washington

Pain Clinic
University of Virginia Medical Center
Charlottesville, Virginia

Pennsylvania Hospital
8th and Spruce Streets
Philadelphia, Pennsylvania
Special orthopedic section for treatment
of back problems.

The Pain Treatment Center
The Johns Hopkins Hospital
Baltimore, Maryland

Pain Treatment Center
Scripps Clinic and Research Foundation
La Jolla, California

The Pain Treatment Center
Montefiore Hospital and Medical Center
Bronx, New York

Rancho Los Amigos Hospital
A unit of the Los Angeles County Hospital System
Downey, California
Rehabilitation of chronic, nonsurgical back problems. Multiphasic treatment approach. Patients encouraged to develop self-health care.

Sacramento Medical Center
Sacramento, California
Special Spine Service center for back problems.

St. Joseph's Hospital
San Francisco, California
Progressive exercise program designed to get the patient functional and back to work as soon as possible. Classes in preventive care and self-healing.

# Sports Medicine Clinics

Center for Sports Medicine and Sciences
Temple University School of Medicine
Philadelphia, Pennsylvania

Department of Orthopedic Surgery
and Sports Medicine
The Cleveland Clinic Foundation
Cleveland, Ohio

Denver Sports Medicine Clinic
2045 Franklin St.
Denver, Colorado

Hughston Orthopedic Clinic
105 Physicians Building
Columbus, Georgia

Institute of Sports Medicine
and Athletic Trauma
Lenox Hill Hospital
New York, New York

National Athletic Health Institute
575 E. Hardy St.
Inglewood, California

National Jogging Association
1910 K Street, N.W., Suite 202
Washington D.C. 20006
You can write in your running health questions
for reply.

Sports Medicine Clinic
Northwestern Medical School
Chicago, Illinois

Sports Medicine Clinic
University of Oklahoma Medical Center
Oklahoma City, Oklahoma

Sports Medicine Resource, Inc.
830 Boylston St.
Chestnut Hill, Massachusetts

Sports Medicine Section,
Division of Orthopedic Surgery
University of Wisconsin Hospitals
Madison, Wisconsin

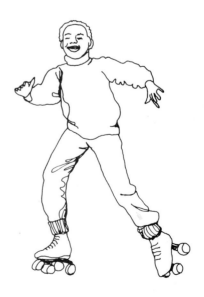

# Glossary

*Acute:* Sudden, sharp, and short.

*The Alexander Technique* is a subtle system of postural alignment which focuses on spinal alignment and movement dynamics.

*Allopathy:* Medical practice which uses remedies to produce effects different from those that the disease being treated causes.

*Animus:* The image toward which we strive, the soul, the spirit, the breath. Also: the male archetype in a woman (as the anima is the female archetype in a man). Also: hostility.

*Articulation:* A loose joining together of parts which allows movement between them.

*Bandage Addiction:* A compulsion to wear bandages even after a wound is healed and a dressing is no longer needed. One sufferer is said to have rebandaged himself daily for twenty-two years.

*Biofeedback:* A training technique which enables individuals to gain some voluntary control over autonomic body functions.

*Breyer Technique:* Doris Breyer is a European therapist working in San Francisco. Her work is a combination of movement, verbal work, and contact alignment. A "therapists' therapist", she is distinguished for having developed work which has had a major influence on the practice of many of the currently prominent therapy experts. Her work is gentle and powerful and unique.

*Bursa:* A membrane-lined sac containing synovial fluid; found or formed in places subject to friction, where tendons pass over bones, for example.

*Bursitis:* an inflammation of the bursa.

*Chakra* is the Indian name for an energy center in the body. The Oriental chakras correspond with Western nerve pulse centers. Each chakra is said to be the seat of a different kind of power.

*Chronic:* long-lasting or recurrent.

*Contusion:* a bruise.

*Cramp:* a painful spasm or temporary muscle paralysis resulting from overexertion.

*Enzymes:* Proteins, produced by cells, which catalyze chemical reactions in other substances without being essentially changed themselves.

*Erector spinae:* deep back muscles which run from the sacral to the lumbar region, then branch in three columns which are attached to the ribs and vertebrae. Their contraction straightens the spinal column.

*Feldenkrais Technique:* Moshe Feldenkrais, a therapist living a Israel, is known for his excellent body therapy techniques which produce dramatic postural realignment through very gentle, subtle body manipulation. He and Ruthy Alon, a Feldenkrais practicioner, travel extensively doing workshops in this method.

*Flexion:* being bent or flexed.

*Gland:* a cell or group of cells that selectively removes certain substances from the blood and alters or concentrates their use in or elimination from the body.

*Hamstrings:* the tendons at the back of the knee.

*Herniated:* ruptured; protruding through an abnormal opening.

*Homeopathy:* medical practice which administers small doses of remedies which in healthy people would produce the effects of the disease under treatment.

*Laminectomy:* surgical removal of the back of the vertebra.

*Ligaments:* bands or sheets of fibrous tissue which connect bones or cartilages, or support muscles or fascia.

*Lumbar Lordosis:* saddle back, hollow back.

*Metabolism:* all the chemical changes which effect nutrition.

*Metastasis:* the shifting of a disease, or its local manifestation from one body part to another; in cancer, the appearance of new growths at sites remote from the primary tumor.

*Muscle tone:* a normal tension which keeps tissues in shape and ready for action.

*Neuritis:* the inflammation of a nerve.

*Occipatal:* relating to the occiput, the bone which forms the back of the skull and is joined to the atlas vertebra.

*Osteoporosis:* a weakening of the bones which occurs in elderly men and menopausal women.

*Polarity Therapy:* a healing system organized by Dr. Randolph Stone, physician to a yogi in India. Polarity is a combination of acupuncture point stimulation, dietary cleansing and postural exercise.

*Psoas Major:* a muscle which runs from the thoracic and lumbar vertebrae to the thigh bone and which flexes the thigh.

*Quadricips:* the great extensor, or straightening muscle of the front of the thigh; attached at four places within the thigh and at the kneecap.

*Rectus Abdominis:* a straight muscle of the abdomen which runs from the pubic bone to the chest.

*Reichian Therapy:* Wilhelm Reich was a European therapist who developed a system of breathing and movement therapy designed to release rigid body structures and personality traits. He is noted for combining his therapy with an analysis of the relationship of body structure to political structure. He was a brilliant theorist who was persecuted in Europe and the U.S. for his anti-fascist stance. Modern day therapies draw heavily on his practices.

*Rolfing:* Ida Rolf was a doctor from Germany who organized an old physical therapy technique, deep tissue massage, into a system of postural realignment. Rolfing is distinct for its use of extremely deep pressure, often painful.

*Sacroiliac:* relating to the sacrum (the vertebrae which are the back wall of the pelvic basin) and the ilia, the upper back sides of the pelvis.

*Sciatic:* in the vicinity of the hips.

*Sciatica:* pain in the sciatic nerve, lower back, buttocks, or hips, usually caused by a herniated lumbar disc, sometimes by sciatic neuritis.

*Scoliosis:* swayback, lateral curvature of the spine.

*Spasm:* an abnormal and involuntary muscle contraction; muscle tension which cannot be released voluntarily.

*Spinabifida:* a defect of the spinal column; the absence of vertebral arches which allows the spinal membrane, and sometimes the spinal cord, to protrude.

*Spondylolisthesis:* slipping forward of a lower lumbar vertebra.

*Sprain:* a joint injury which may involve the rupture of tendons or ligaments but no fracture or dislocation.

*Spurs:* dull spines or projections from bones.

*Statics:* the mechanics of the relations of forces which produce equilibrium.

*Strain:* just what it sounds like; an injury resulting from overuse, improper use, or excessive pressure.

*Toxin:* a poison produced by metabolism.

*Traction:* a pulling force; in medicine, a technique of using weights to pull limbs in suspension in an attempt to alleviate pressure and align muscles and bones.

# Notes

1. Milne, A.A. POOH'S BIRTHDAY BOOK. E.P. Dutton, 1963.

2. Plato. CHARMIDES. c. 399 B.C.

3. Constitution of the World Health Organization, PREAMBLE, 1946.

4. Flynn, Errol. MY WICKED, WICKED WAYS. Putnam, 1959.

5. Storm, Hyemeyohsts. SEVEN ARROWS. Ballantine, 1972.

6. Oelbaum, Cynthia H. *American Journal of Nursing*, 1974.

7. Winter, Nina. INTERVIEW WITH THE MUSE. Moon Books, 1978.

8. Woolf, Virginia. A ROOM OF ONE'S OWN. E.P. Dutton, 1976.

9. Root, Leon, M.D. & Kiernan, Thomas. OH, MY ACHING BACK. Signet, 1973.

10. Ullyot, Dr. Jane. WOMEN'S RUNNING. World, 1976.

11. Leibowitz, Fran. METROPOLITAN LIFE. E.P. Dutton, 1978.

12. Grotjahn, Alfred. SOCIAL HYGIENE. 1847.

13. Dew, Joan. SINGERS AND SWEETHEARTS. Doubleday, 1977.

14. Finneson, Bernard, M.D. THE NEW APPROACH TO LOW BACK PAIN. Berkley, 1975.

15. Root, Leon, M.D. (see note 9).

16. Mead, Margaret. NEW REALITIES MAGAZINE; Vol. II #2, 1978.

17. Waley, Arthur. THE NINE SONGS OF SHAMANISM IN ANCIENT CHINA. City Lights Books, 1973.

18. Root, Leon, M.D. (see note 9).

19. Lettvin, Maggie. MAGGIE'S BACK BOOK. Houghton Mifflin, 1976.

20. Mitchell, Yvonne. COLETTE: A TASTE FOR LIFE. Harcourt Brace Jovanovich, 1975.

---

Many thanks to David Shiang for his fine proofreading.

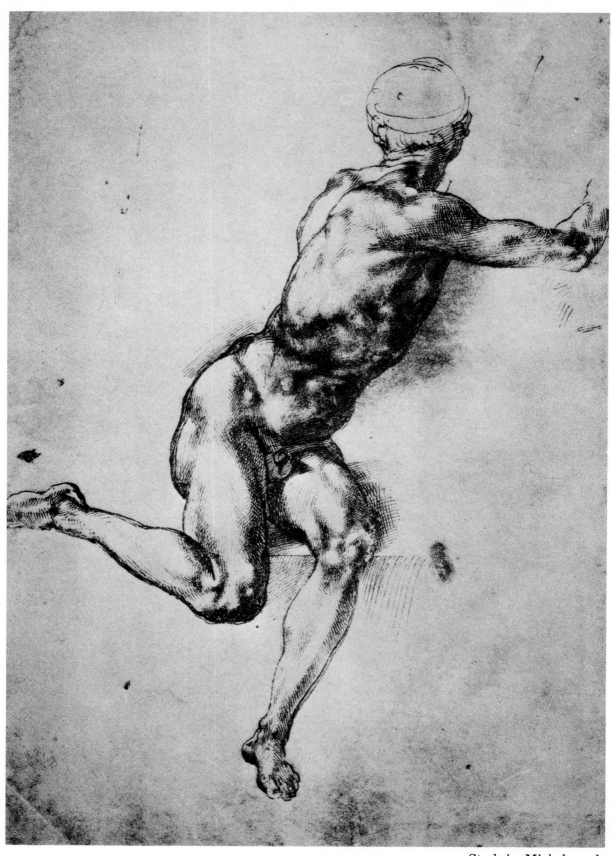

Study by **Michelangelo**

# Bibliography

Alexander, F. Matthias. THE RESURRECTION OF THE BODY. Delta, 1971.

Back Pain Association Limited. *Talkback*. A newsletter intended to disseminate information relevant to the field of back pain. Grundy House, Somerset Road, Teddington, Middlesex TW11 8TD England.

Beals, Rodney and Hickman, Norman. "Industrial Injuries of the Back and Extremities." *Journal of Bone and Joint Surgery*. Vol. 54-A, No. 8, Dec., 1972.

Beau, Georges, CHINESE MEDICINE. Avon, 1965.

Blumenthal, Lester. "Injury to the Cervical Spine as a Cause of Headache." *Postgraduate Medicine*. Vol. 56, No. 3, Sept., 1974.

"Biofeedback: A Demand for Clinical Expertise." *Texas Medicine*, Vol. 71, No. 3, Sept., 1975.

Brown, Isadore. "Intensive Exercises for the Low Back." *Physical Therapy*. Vol. 50, No. 4, April, 1970.

Campbell, Joseph. THE MYSTERIES. Bollingen Series, Princeton University Press, 1955.

Cerney, J.V. ACUPUNCTURE WITHOUT NEEDLES. Parker Publishing Co., Inc., 1974.

Cerney, J.V. HANDBOOK OF UNUSUAL AND UNORTHODOX HEALING METHODS. Parker Publishing Co., Inc., 1976.

Chamberlain, Geoffrey. "Backache II." *British Medical Journal*. April 17, 1971.

Chang, Jolan. THE TAO OF LOVE AND SEX. E.P. Dutton, 1977.

Chesler, Phyllis. WOMEN AND MADNESS. Doubleday, 1972.

Cooper, Kenneth, M.D. THE NEW AEROBICS. Bantam, 1970.

Corea, Gena. THE HIDDEN MALPRACTICE: HOW AMERICAN MEDICINE MISTREATS WOMEN. Jove-Harcourt Brace Jovanovich, 1978.

Cyriax, James. THE SLIPPED DISC. Gower Press, 1975.

Daly, Mary. GYN/ECOLOGY: THE META-ETHICS OF RADICAL FEMINISM. Beacon Press, 1978.

Ehrenreich, Barbara and English, Deidre. FOR HER OWN GOOD. Anchor, 1978.

Eliade, Mircea. FROM PRIMITIVES TO ZEN. Harper & Row, 1977.

Feldenkrais, Moshe. AWARENESS THROUGH MOVEMENT. Harper & Row, 1972.

Finneson, Bernard and Freese, Arthur. THE NEW APPROACH TO LOW BACK PAIN. Berkley Publishing Corp., 1975.

# BIBLIOGRAPHY

Friedman, Lawrence and Galton, Lawrence. FREEDOM FROM BACKACHES. Simon & Schuster, Inc., 1973.

Garrett, J.F. and Ahmad, Irshad. "The Industrial Back Problem: Role of the Industrial Hygienist and Ergonomics." American Industrial Hygiene Association. Vol. 38, No. 10, Oct., 1977.

Gauquelin, Michel. COSMIC CLOCKS. Henry Regnery Co., 1967.

Gottlieb, Harold, *et. al.* "Comprehensive Rehabilitation of Patients Having Chronic Low Back Pain." Archives of Physical Medicine Rehabilitation. Vol. 58, March, 1977.

Gould, Heywood. HEADACHES: CAUSES, TREATMENT AND PREVENTION. Barnes & Noble Books, 1973.

Hopkins, Henry, M.D. LEOPOLD'S PRINCIPLES AND METHODS OF PHYSICAL DIAGNOSIS. W.B. Saunders Co., 1966.

Horter, Tracy. "How To Care for Your Neck." *Physical Therapy.* Vol. 58, No. 2, Feb., 1978.

Illich, Ivan. MEDICAL NEMESIS. Bantam, 1977.

Jaynes, Julian. THE ORIGIN OF CONSCIOUSNESS IN THE BREAKDOWN OF THE BICAMERAL MIND. Houghton Mifflin, 1976.

Kendall, Henry O. and Kendall, Florence P. "Developing and Maintaining Good Posture." PHYSICAL THERAPY. Vol. 48, No. 4, April, 1968.

Kramos. Paul. "New Rules Fight Back Injuries." INTERNATIONAL JOURNAL OF OCCUPATIONAL HEALTH AND SAFETY. Vol. 41, Sept-Oct., 1975.

Kraus, Hans. "Prevention of Low Back Pain." *Journal of Occupational Medicine.* Nov., 1967.

Krupp, Marcus, M.D., *et. al.* PHYSICIAN'S HANDBOOK. Lange Medical Publications. 1973.

Kurland, Howard. "Treatment of Headache Pain with Auto-Accupressure." *Diseases of the Nervous System.* Vol. 37, March, 1975.

Kurland, Howard, M.D. QUICK HEADACHE RELIEF WITHOUT DRUGS. Ballantine, 1977.

Leavitt, Frank; Garron, David; Whisler, Walter; Sheinkop, Mitchell. "Affective and Sensory Dimensions of Back Pain." PAIN. 1978.

Lettvin, Allan. "Surgical Treatment of Low Back Pain." *Nursing Times.* Nov. 7, 1974.

Lettvin, Maggie. MAGGIE'S BACK BOOK. Houghton Mifflin, 1976.

Luce, Gay Gaer. BODY TIME. Pantheon, 1971.

Mann, Felix. ACUPUNCTURE—THE ANCIENT ART OF HEALING. Vintage, 1972.

Mantle, M.J.; Greenwood, R.M., and Currey, H.L.F. "Backache in Pregnancy." *Rheumatology and Rehabilitation.* Vol. 16, 1977.

Mastrovito, Rene C. "Psychogenic Pain." *American Journal of Nursing.* March, 1974.

Mookerjee, Ajit. TANTRA ART. Kumar Gallery, New Delhi, 1966.

Navarro, Vicente. MEDICINE UNDER CAPITALISM. Prodist Publications, 1976.

Nomadic Sisters. LOVING WOMEN. Nomadic Sisters, 1975.

Oelbaum, Cynthia Hastings. "Hallmarks of Adult Wellness." *American Journal of Nursing.* Vol. 74. No. 9, Sept., 1974.

Oyle, Irving. THE HEALING MIND. Celestial Arts, 1975.

Pawl, Ronald. "Headache, Cervical Spondylosis and Anterior Cervical Fusion." SURGERY ANNUAL. 1977.

Pick, Pickering and Howden, Robert, eds. GRAY'S ANATOMY. Running Press, 1977.

Pos, Robert. "Psychological Assessment of Factors Affecting Pain." *Canadian Medical Association Journal.* Vol. 3, Dec. 7, 1974.

Prevention Magazine Staff. THE ENCYCLOPEDIA OF COMMON DISEASES. Rodale Press, 1976.

Reiter, Rayna R., ed. TOWARD AN ANTHROPOLOGY OF WOMEN. Monthly Review Press, 1975.

Revolutionary Health Committee of Hunan Province. A BAREFOOT DOCTOR'S MANUAL. Cloudburst Press, 1977.

Rich, Adrienne. OF WOMAN BORN. Bantam, 1977.

Root, Leon, M.D., and Kierman, Thomas. OH, MY ACHING BACK. Signet, 1973.

Rose, Jeanne. KITCHEN COSMETICS. Panjandrum/Aris Books, 1978.

Rowan, Robert, M.D. and Gillette, Paul. THE GAY HEALTH GUIDE. Little, Brown & Co., 1978.

Rubin, David. "The No! Or the Yes and How—Of Sex for Patients with Neck, Back and Radicular Pain Syndromes." *California Medicine.* Vol. 113, No. 6, Dec., 1970.

Simons, Gene and Mirabile, Mathew. "An Analysis and Interpretation of Industrial Medical Data: With Concentration on Back Problems." *Journal of Occupational Medicine.* Vol. 14, No. 3, March, 1972.

Smith, Clyde F. "Physical Management of Muscular Low Back Pain." *Canadian Medical Assoc. Journal.* Vol. 117, No. 6, Sept. 17, 1977.

STEDMAN'S MEDICAL DICTIONARY. Williams & Wilkins Co., 1976.

Sternback, Richard, *et al.* "Aspects of Chronic Low Back Pain."*Psychosomatics.* Vol. 14, Jan.-Feb., 1973.

Stewart, Elizabeth. "To Lessen Pain: Relaxation and Rhythmic Breathing." *American Journal of Nursing.* June, 1976.

# BIBLIOGRAPHY

Tauber, Joseph. "An Unorthodox Look at Backaches." *Journal of Occupational Medicine.* Vol. 12, April, 1970.

Travell, Janet. "Ladies & Gentlemen, Be Seated Properly." *Reader's Digest.* Aug., 1961.

Turnbull, Sister Joyce. "Shifting the Focus to Health." *American Journal of Nursing.* Dec., 1976.

Ullyot, Joan. WOMEN'S RUNNING. World Publications. 1976.

WET: The Magazine of Gourmet Bathing and Beyond. P.O. Box 1017, Venice, CA. 90291.

White, A.W.M. "Low Back Pain in Men Receiving Workman's Compensation." *Canadian Medical Association Journal.* Vol. 95, July 9, 1966.

"Work Injuries and Illnesses in California Quarterly." Division of Labor Statistics & Research, Nov., 1977.

Zuipema, George, M.D. THE JOHNS HOPKINS ATLAS OF HUMAN FUNCTIONAL ANATOMY. Johns Hopkins University Press, 1977.

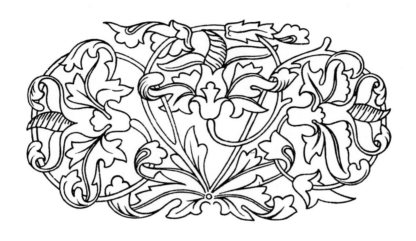

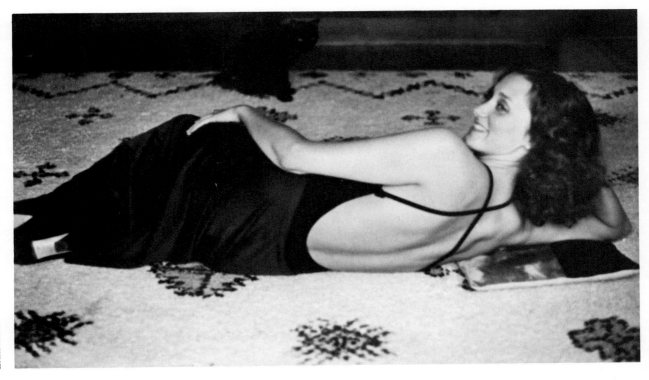

Erika Asher

## The Author

Anne Kent Rush was born in Mobile, Alabama, a descendant of Dr. Benjamin Rush, an American health revolutionary who signed the Declaration of Independence. Rush received her Bachelor's Degree in English from Wayne State University in Detroit, and did post degree studies in etching at the Boston Museum School of Fine Arts. She is the author of GETTING CLEAR: BODY WORK FOR WOMEN (Random House/Bookworks); MOON, MOON (Random House/Moon Books); co-author of FEMINISM AS THERAPY (Random House/Bookworks); and editor and illustrator of THE MASSAGE BOOK (Random House/Bookworks). She was on the training staff of Esalen Institute in California for several years, where she taught doctors and other health professionals how to integrate body therapy into their work. Now Rush runs Moon Books, a publishing house in Berkeley specializing in quality books by women.

The health of all peoples is fundamental to the attainment of peace and security and is dependent upon the fullest cooperation of individuals and States.
—Preamble, United Nations Declaration of Human Rights

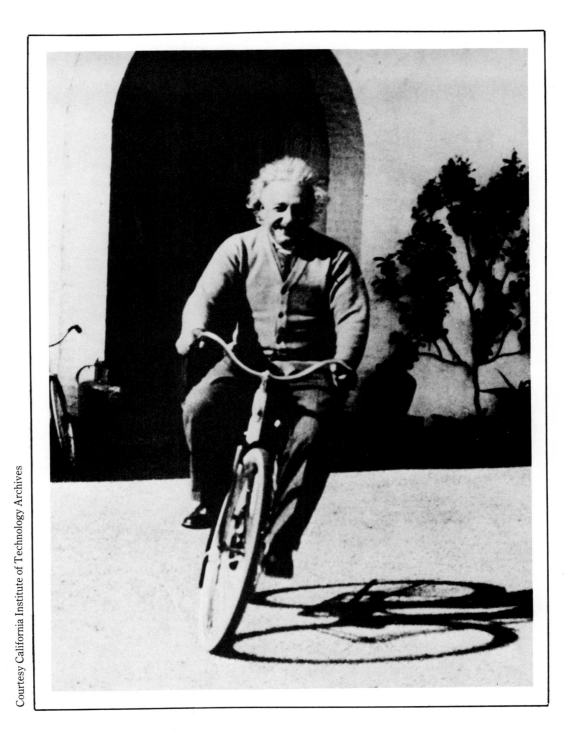

*Albert Einstein,* 1933

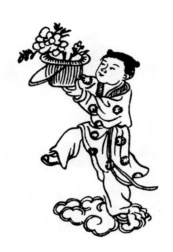

It taught me my most essential art, which is not the art of writing, but the domestic art of knowing how to wait . . . To change the worst into the not so bad. How to lose and recover in the same instant that frivolous thing, a taste for life.[20]

—Colette

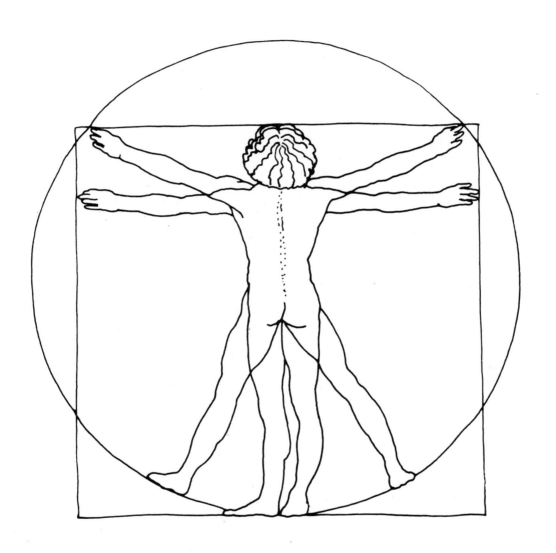

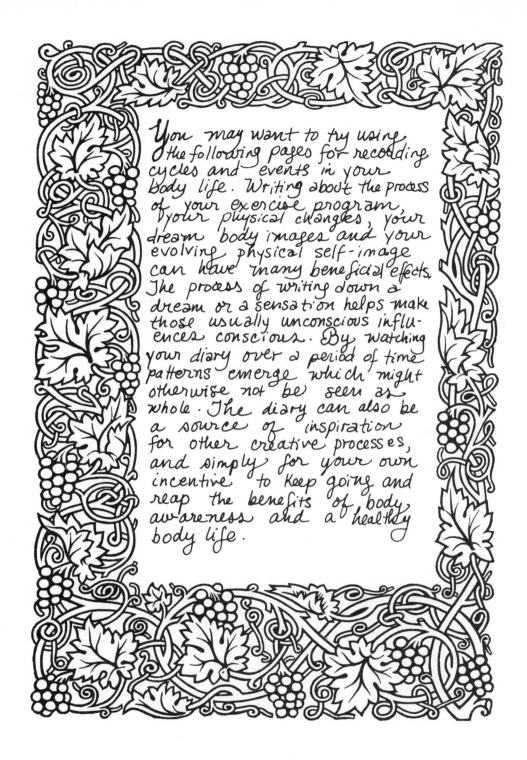

You may want to try using the following pages for recording cycles and events in your body life. Writing about the process of your exercise program, your physical changes, your dream body images and your evolving physical self-image can have many beneficial effects. The process of writing down a dream or a sensation helps make those usually unconscious influences conscious. By watching your diary over a period of time patterns emerge which might otherwise not be seen as whole. The diary can also be a source of inspiration for other creative processes, and simply for your own incentive to keep going and reap the benefits of body awareness and a healthy body life.

BODY LIFE DIARY